THE HOSPICE

Development and Administration

Edited by

GLEN W. DAVIDSON

Southern Illinois University, Springfield

HEMISPHERE
PUBLISHING CORPORATION
Washington   New York   London

THE HOSPICE: Development and Administration

3 4 5 6 7 8 9 0   B R B R   7 8 3 2 1 0 9

Library of Congress Cataloging in Publication Data
Main entry under title:

The Hospice: development and administration.

    Bibliography: p.
    Includes index.
    1. Terminal care. 2. Terminal care facilities.
I. Davidson, Glen W. [DNLM: 1. Hospitals, Special—
North America. 2. Terminal care. 3. Death. WB27 DA2
H8]
R726.8.H66   362.1'9'6   78-3836
ISBN 0-89116-103-1

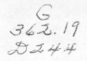

∞∞∞

CONTENTS

∞∞∞

ISSUES IN CARING

ANNOTATIONS

PREFACE

So far as can be determined, this is the first attempt to bring together in one volume a report on the hospice movement in North America. This book covers what has occurred and what is being planned for better institutional care of the terminally ill.

Dying and living in the face of death are not new. Nor is caring for the terminally ill. Like other aspects of "mass society," comprehensive health care has, even while offering better and more widespread services, so disrupted traditional rituals of care known by our parents that this generation has had to radically reexamine how best to preserve human dignity in the closing moments of life. We have not only the opportunity to bring to the care of the terminally ill new medications, new skills, and new understanding, but also the obligation to restore a unified, "wholistic" approach to terminal care.

Hospice is a medieval term, referring to the wayside inns for pilgrims and other travelers, particularly at those places of greatest vulnerability and hardship. Much of the inspiration for the hospice movement in North America has been provided by Dr. Cicely Saunders, who founded St. Christopher's Hospice in London. Like all other European institutions brought to this continent, however, unique needs and values have reshaped, reorganized, and reapplied the original vision.

This volume is organized into four sections. The six hospice or palliative care programs described in the first section are not the first institutions in North America to be concerned with specialized care of the dying. Some of the first "hospitals" established in 17th century New France and New England appear to have had no other reason for existence than terminal care. Various religious communities in both Canada and the United States have long supported palliative care facilities of which the most famous is probably Calvary Hospital in the Bronx, now being modernized through a massive rebuilding scheme.

What the six programs do represent is the effort to approach the needs of terminally ill patients, their families, and the staffs who tend them with a renewed sense of compassion like that achieved at St. Christopher's Hospice. None of the programs is exactly like St. Christopher's. All have developed out of the identified needs and possibilities of specific locations.

As a quick glance at the Directory of Hospice Programs in this book will show, the six programs do not begin to represent all the ways institutional care can be organized. It is hoped, however, that from the descriptions of these six programs—all at different points of development—the reader can see how the hospice movement in North America is taking shape.

The second section discusses problems when caring for the terminally ill. The unquestioned assumption in the hospice movement is that staff who care for the terminally ill must be specially trained and oriented if this care is to be different from that given in a hospital or nursing home. Staff stress is the most frequently mentioned problem with hospice services.

The essays in this section include Sr. Simone Roach's attempt to find a different approach to the educational process from that found in many training programs for nursing staff members. Mary Vachon and colleagues from The Clarke Institute, who have written the most extensive study of staff stress, identify possible motivations for giving care to the terminally ill, which in turn may lead to high stress among staff members. Barry Rogers addresses patient stress from the perspective of thwarted creativity and describes an approach in creative communications used at Hill-haven Hospice. Robert Buckingham and Susan Foley describe some of the problems of evaluating whether a program is delivering the quality of care desired.

The third section looks at some of the basic issues of hospice care. Conspicuously missing is an essay on issues of funding hospice programs. Difficulties in funding have tended to dominate discussions about, and workshops on, hospice care. Economics are very important. But basic principles of care too frequently are prostituted for the sake of bureaucratic whims—"fiscal account-ability"—and the issues of *whether* hospice programs should be funded and *what* characteristics of care should be given emphasis are obscured. Assumptions about "dignity" are among the obscurities. Using the concept of dignity as an entrance into some of the issues of hospice care, three essays raise questions from "spiritual," ethical, and legal perspectives.

The final section is intended to assist those readers who want to know more about hospice programs or who want assistance with their own development of hospice services. Parimala Desai has selected references in health care literature largely from journals published since 1970. Richard Dayringer comments on use of audiovisual materials for training staff in patient care. The Directory of Hospice Programs is incomplete but is the most up-to-date that can be provided the reader at this time.

Like all basic functions of life, each generation must relearn how human beings can best survive, not just physically, but in that whole realm we call *living*. What seems to be new in the hospice movement in North America is the sense that for this generation, compassion does not need to be sacrificed for economic, professional, technocratic, or scientific reasons. This volume is only a beginning on how the critically and terminally ill, their families, and the staff who care for them wrestle with questions of care, competence, and compassion.

Glen W. Davidson

MODELS OF CARE

∞∞

MONTREAL (1975)—THE ROYAL VICTORIA HOSPITAL PALLIATIVE CARE SERVICE

∞∞

DOTTIE C. WILSON, INA AJEMIAN, and
BALFOUR M. MOUNT
Royal Victoria Hospital
Montreal, Quebec, Canada

The Palliative Care Service was developed after staff at the Royal Victoria Hospital, a McGill University teaching hospital, identified serious deficiencies in care of terminally ill patients and their families. The service, including both an in-hospital unit and a home care program, cares for patients for whom treatment aimed at cure or prolongation of life is no longer appropriate. Its multidisciplinary team aims to meet the medical, psychological, social, and spiritual needs of patients and their families.

Introduction

"If it can be done at the Royal Victoria Hospital it can be done anywhere!" This observation from one of our colleagues regarding a palliative care service may not be entirely accurate. Indeed, many key factors came together to make it particularly opportune in that place, at that time. His words do, however, serve to emphasize the significant fact that a major university teaching hospital, whose reputation was established through basic research, teaching, and skilled tertiary care, has fostered the development of a new type of service whose goals, philosophy, and daily routines stand in stark contrast to the traditional medical model and standards of the institution. In many aspects the experiment was without precedent. On innumerable occasions the comforting excellence and success of St. Christopher's Hospice in London seemed almost mocking. Ours was a different cultural setting. Furthermore, our attempts would find us not in a secluded haven where we could develop in safety, but at the very center of an institution that epitomizes the medical information explosion and expanding technology. The details concerning this odyssey from germinal idea to busy service are set forth here in the hope that they may be of some use to others embarking on a similar journey.

Examining the Need

In February 1973, one of us was asked to participate in a panel discussion on the subject of death and dying. He was invited because he was a physician and not because of any particular interest in the field at that time.

In preparing for this discussion with other panel members, the following questions were raised. What are the needs of the terminally ill? Are those persons supplying health care fulfilling these needs? As we do not seem to know, how can we find out? These questions led to the organization of the Ad Hoc Committee on Thanatology at the Royal Victoria Hospital. The objectives of this multidisciplinary committee were to:

1. Determine the emotional and physical needs of the terminally ill at the hospital.
2. Identify areas of deficiency in meeting these needs.
3. Explore possible solutions for identified deficiencies.

A research grant of $2,000 was awarded to the committee by McGill University. Steps taken to achieve these objectives were to:

1. Construct a multiple choice questionnaire.
2. Conduct an opinion survey regarding attitudes of patients and hospital staff toward terminal illness.
3. Develop in-depth case studies of selected patients.
4. Consult with Dr. Elisabeth Kübler-Ross.
5. Visit St. Christopher's Hospice in London, England.

In an effort to determine how the hospital staff and its terminally ill patients felt about death and the emotional needs of the dying, a questionnaire was devised and circulated to all members of the attending staff—residents and interns, nurses, social workers, physical and occupational therapists, and clergy—as well as selected terminally ill patients.

Approximately 1,600 questionnaires were distributed. They were mailed in the intrahospital system to resident and attending staff physicians, while all nurses received the questionnaire from their head nurse or with their paychecks. Members of the clergy, social workers, physiotherapists, and occupational therapists were given their questionnaires individually. Each questionnaire was accompanied by a brief explanatory letter, earnestly requesting cooperation and signed by the medical director, chairman of the medical board, and director of nursing (in the case of nurses). A return envelope was enclosed, addressed to the office of the medical director, to facilitate the anonymous completion and return of the questionnaire.

Patients were selected for interview on the basis of two criteria: (1) Their illness was of sufficient consequence to have led them, probably, at some point to consider their own demise, and (2) their physician did not object to the interview. The interviewer, a second-year medical student, was the same for all patients. Following an explanation that we at the Royal Victoria Hospital wish to learn from our patients about how we can better meet their needs, the questionnaire was reviewed and answered by the patient with the assistance of the interviewer.

The format of the questionnaire was determined by the following principles:

1. "Hard" data would be desirable although the "soft" subjective nature of the topic would make it necessary to adopt artificial and rigid generalizations to attain this end.
2. All groups should be asked the same questions to facilitate data analysis and highlight the problem areas.
3. Questions should aim at asking the participants: (a) Is there a problem? (b) How do they respond to the issues personally? (c) How do their colleagues respond to them? (d) How do those in other professions respond?

In addition to age, sex, marital status, religion, and profession, 21 multiple choice questions were asked. Prior to completion of the protocol, a restricted trial run was made to assist with refining the wording of the questions. Several changes were made.

The data received (1) indicated that (a) patients desired complete openness and honesty in discussion of diagnosis and prognosis, (b) physicians were reluctant to be that candid, (c) residents seemed to lack concern for the patients' emotional needs, and (d) social workers tended to minimize the problem. Physicians' attitudes toward their own deaths were found to be an important variable in determining how they perceived patients' needs: 85 percent of the physicians who felt they would want to know their own prognosis if they were fatally ill thought that their patients also desired direct communication of prognosis, while only 45 percent of the physicians not wanting to know their own prognosis thought their patients desired honest communication.

The data indicated that in each professional group the proportion who recognized deficiencies in the way in which their colleagues met the needs of the terminally ill was larger than the proportion who recognized that they themselves had deficiencies. Similarly, the proportion who felt that they personally avoided discussion with patients regarding dying was smaller than the proportion who felt that their colleagues avoided such discussions. It was also noted that patients are reluctant to criticize those who care for them.

The Report of the Ad Hoc Committee on Thanatology was presented to the executive committee, medical advisory board, and the attending staff of the hospital in the autumn of 1973. This report provided a body of data so persuasive it could not be ignored. The demonstration of local problems and the potential creative solutions such as seen at St. Christopher's Hospice were important factors.

It was indisputably clear that the hospital was deficient in meeting the needs of the terminally ill. The recommendation that a hospice unit or palliative care unit be established to better meet these needs was a natural outcome of the compiled data. It is to the credit of the hospital that when the problem was identified, the recommended solution was adopted.

Rationale

Why should there be a separate unit in a general hospital? Why not educate all hospital staff?

While recent educational programs in death and dying have increased hospital staff awareness of the particular needs of terminally ill patients and their families, there remains a basic problem. The training and skills of professional staff in a general hospital are focused toward four ends: investigation, diagnosis, cure, and prolongation of life. These activities are largely irrelevant to terminally ill patients, for whom quality of life is the only appropriate focus. To maintain that the staff of acute-care wards should fully meet the needs of this patient group is to ignore the pressures of medical "future shock" that are already on them. We cannot be all things to all people. Sustained excellence demands that the health care team have particular expertise in the area of their patients' needs.

Why have a unit in a general hospital instead of a separate institution? Being part of a general hospital provides a variety of advantages:

1. It avoids the building of new palliative care facilities in a community that cannot afford sufficient new beds to meet the needs of the 70 percent of North Americans dying in institutions.
2. The close proximity of palliative and acute-care units may stimulate improved quality of care in both programs.
3. It facilitates the use of existing general hospital resources including skilled personnel and equipment (e.g., radiation therapy) when needed for palliation.
4. It enables the hospital that cares for patients in all other phases of life to meet its responsibility to them when they are dying.

Obtaining Support

The Palliative Care Unit was opened in January 1975 after a further 15 months of intense, continuing pressure for space, funding, and support. Steps taken included the following:

1. The committee's findings were presented at grand rounds in the Departments of Medicine, Surgery, Obstetrics and Gynecology, Urology, and Psychiatry. This aided in mobilizing the support of the attending staff.
2. Further hard data were collected concerning (a) inpatient cancer deaths during the previous 3 years, (b) inpatient terminal cancer days over the same period (24–32 days), and (c) the number of terminal patients referred to social service for placement during this period.

These data helped determine the patient pool and the number of beds required. A series of events followed before the opening of the unit in January 1975:

First, a presentation was made to a private philanthropic organization using the committee report data. Its grant of $100,000 over 3 years, commencing September 1974, enabled preliminary research, detailed planning, and building of a multidisciplinary team to precede the opening of the unit.

Second, after Dr. Kübler-Ross visited and gave a public address at the hospital to an overflow audience, the pressure increased.

Third, a large newspaper spread concerning the Committee's findings added public interest, as did other media presentations and personal talks in the community.

Fourth, a Core Group was formed that met to discuss the details of how the service would function. This group included physicians, a social worker, nurses, a chaplain representative, a dietician, and an administrator. Minutes of these meetings were circulated to the hospital administration.

Fifth, because decisions to suspend "active treatment" must be made by nonpalliative care physicians to avoid conflict-of-interest charges, a Physicians Advisory Committee was formed, made up of consultants in the various related fields of medical, surgical and gynecologic oncology, radiotherapy, and anesthesiology.

Sixth, key staff members gained important experience at St. Christopher's Hospice.

Seventh, in the final months of 1974 a team of approximately 50 volunteers was developed after a process of careful screening and comprehensive training.

Even though there was a serious nursing shortage in the province of Quebec at that time, the philosophy of palliative care attracted enough nurses to the hospital to enable the opening of a 12-bed unit. The unit was established as a 2-year pilot project to determine the feasibility of such a service in a general hospital.

The Palliative Care Service

The Palliative Care Service is concerned with four areas of care: an in-patient facility (the *Palliative Care Unit*), a hospital-based *home care program,* a *consultation team,* and a *bereavement follow-up group.* Research, teaching, and administration are also important functions of the service.

During the 2-year pilot project phase, the patient pool was limited to Royal Victoria Hospital patients with malignant diseases for whom care aimed at improving the quality of life was the only appropriate therapy. It was understood that as the unit increased in size, patients with other diseases would be considered.

The Palliative Care Unit

The Palliative Care Unit admits only patients for whom cure and prolongation of life are no longer appropriate goals, whose referring physician has decided on the transfer. The decision to admit a patient is made by the palliative care physician and the head nurse. An admissions committee periodically reviews admission criteria and is consulted for special problems. Priority for admission has been given to:

1. Patients difficult to manage in other departments because of poorly controlled physical symptoms or difficult psychosocial situations.
2. Patients in the home care program requiring admission.

While the patient may be admitted under the name of the referring doctor for reimbursement purposes, day-to-day management is directed, and all orders written, by the unit physician. The referring physician is encouraged to continue his involvement as a consultant.

If the admission is a transfer from another ward in the hospital, the patient or a family member is invited to visit the unit prior to the transfer. This does a great deal to reassure anxious patients. At the time of transfer, a staff member goes to the floor to accompany the patient to the unit.

On direct admissions from home, the patient is brought straight to the unit on arrival at the hospital. Only after the patient is settled and comfortable does the family go to the admitting office to complete necessary forms. The goal of admission procedure is to give the patient a sense of welcome to a place where people care for the patient as an individual and to work to relieve any distress. Use of personal name cards, greetings by name, and bedside flowers are part of the unit's style of operation. Both patient and family are familiarized with ward routines and the family is reassured that they can continue to be involved in the patient's care to whatever degree they feel comfortable. There are no "visiting hour" restrictions and no age minimum for visitors. A family member may stay overnight if need arises. A pet may visit if it is important to the patient. The family is encouraged to bring in the patient's favorite foods— there is a microwave oven, refrigerator, etc. for preparing meals and snacks.

Palliative care means symptom control (2, p. 66; 3, 4) achieved by a health care team skilled in clinical pharmacology. Many patients with advanced malignant diseases have heard their medical team say, verbally or nonverbally, "there is nothing more that can be done." Those working in palliative care must declare in action that there is much that can and must be done. The physical, social, psychological, and spiritual components of "total pain" must be attacked in the context of a supportive milieu including family and unit staff. Patient and family together are considered the focus of care. Care is given by a multidisciplinary team made up of physicians, nurses and nursing aides, social worker, ward clerk, dietician, physiotherapist, chaplains, recreational therapist, music therapist, and volunteers.

As death approaches, the attention of the team is focused on giving maximum reassurance and comfort to patient and family. When death has occurred, the family is encouraged to grieve at bedside in a viewing room located in the unit.

A patient may be sent home if his symptoms can be brought under control and if patient and family feel able to cope. They are followed by the home care nurse and are assured of readmission if the need should arise.

Home Care Program

The home care team accepts patients on the same basis as the unit. In addition, when patient load permits, the team may follow patients who are still undergoing active treatment for prolongation of life. In this case, the referring physician continues to supervise the active treatment while the palliative care physician is in charge of pain and symptom control. Should such a patient require hospital admission, it is to the referring doctor's service, not to the palliative care unit. The home care team also follows patients who are discharged home from the Palliative Care Unit.

The home care staff at present consists of four nurses and a physician. They cover nights and weekends on rotation to supply 24-hour coverage. In addition, volunteers, the physiotherapist, and the social worker make home visits and are involved in home-care patient and family problems when the need arises. Coordination of community resources is the joint responsibility of home-care nurses and the social worker.

As in the unit, home care includes controlling pain and symptoms as well as seeking resolution of emotional, interpersonal, spiritual, and financial difficulties. Families may phone the unit any time there is a problem, and patients are admitted when the family can no longer cope.

The Consultation Team

Patients are seen in consultation at the request of their attending physician or the ward staff concerned. The Palliative Care Service physician and consultation nurse assist the referring ward in development of a comprehensive care plan, which may include transfer to the unit or to home care.

Since the Palliative Care Service cannot care for all terminally ill patients in the hospital, teaching philosophy and skills of palliative care to other staff is a key priority. Within the hospital, teaching is carried out by the consultation nurse and the palliative care physicians. The consultation nurse participates in regular group discussions with nursing staff throughout the hospital, discussing general principles of palliative care or difficulties of a specific patient. The most significant teaching frequently takes place on a one-to-one basis as the consultation team works on other floors and as staff there witness an improvement in patient/family care as a result of the new care plan. The plan includes bereavement follow-up. A small team of carefully selected volunteers is used for this work.

Bereavement Follow-up

Bereavement represents a period of crisis. In the Palliative Care Service, families are encouraged to acknowledge the realities of impending loss. Members of the team are supportive, and open to discuss and assist with anticipatory grief.

Key family members particularly close to the patient (key persons) are assessed prospectively for risk of impairment of health and psychosocial adjustment. Those considered at risk are followed and those not at risk may or may not be followed by the Palliative Care Service staff after the death of the patient.

Follow-up includes telephone contact 2 weeks after the death, a visit by a staff member—usually a nurse close to the family during the admission—at approximately 1 month, and a letter 1 year later. More extensive follow-up is available when indicated. Home care staff usually follow families of home care patients even though the patient may have been admitted to the unit during the final phase.

Follow-up is carried out under the direction and with the support of the social worker. Bereavement follow-up meetings are held weekly to discuss families visited and the needs seen. These meetings are attended by the social worker and the consultant psychiatrist.

In addition to individual bereavement follow-up activities, family members have been brought together at wine-and-cheese evenings at the hospital. The purpose of these meetings is to share, in an accepting and understanding atmosphere, past and present experiences and feelings with others who are bereaved.

Other Activities

In addition to clinical activity the service has been active in the following:

1. Research and evaluation of our work and of the needs of the terminally ill.
2. Teaching: Continuing education of our own team; participating in McGill's School of Medicine, School of Social Work, School of Nursing, and other courses concerning behavioral sciences and medical ethics; participating in hospital teaching programs and rounds; organizing and participating in conferences and seminars; and offering exposure to and participation in palliative care service activities for visiting health care professionals either on regularly scheduled guest rounds or for a period of 1 month, part of which time is spent working as a nursing assistant on the palliative care unit; and public education through lectures, seminars, and media presentations via television, radio, newspapers, magazines, etc.

Staffing

The needs of terminally ill patients and their families are complex, demanding, and draining. No one person has all the answers or can successfully carry this load unsupported for any significant period of time. The key to success is the use of a highly skilled and experienced multidisciplinary team. Such a team is not fashioned overnight but is molded slowly with careful selection and thoughtful nurturing. Total care is made easier when a variety of personnel with a variety of resources work together. The team approach is not easy, particularly when roles are being redefined from traditional medical models. Members must resolve to break down interprofessional rivalries, set aside defensive attitudes and learn to *know, trust,* and *listen* to each other. Communication is essential and requires both time and effort.

Day-to-day communication in the Palliative Care Service is accomplished through a series of reports and meetings. Information is transmitted also through the use of a communications book, which staff members read each day. In addition, orientation programs, training programs, service rounds, and occasional guest lectures continue in-service education in this field.

Staff support systems include regular meetings, one-to-one conversations between staff members and the consultant psychiatrist, the social worker, or other members of the team. A relaxed informal atmosphere, the presence of children, and the celebration of birthdays and other "live events" are seen as significant factors for supporting staff. Social activities such as staff parties have been held periodically. Such support systems are essential for personnel working in specialized hospital settings where they are under stress of frequent and inevitable patient deaths (5).

The Patient and Key Persons as Team Members

The patient and key persons (family and others at significant risk in bereavement) are integral members of the health care team on the Palliative Care Unit. This fact is symbolic of the differences in direction between palliative and acute care wards. The significance of their inclusion on the team lies not only in the need to consult and obtain active input from them in drawing up the plan of care but also in the need to include them directly as care *givers* (and not just receivers) wherever possible. Such a policy serves to counter the institutional depersonalization many of these patients have experienced. It also assists the key persons in their anticipatory grief.

The inclusion of the patient/family unit on the health care team requires patience and a clear understanding of goals. It represents such a major departure from the usual training of health professionals that frequent refocusing on this issue is required during staff meetings.

The Physicians

The physicians are involved not only in patient care and staff/team support, but also in administration, research, and teaching. A Physician Advisory Committee exists to consult with the medical staff and to relate to the rest of the hospital attending staff. The committee is made up of medical, surgical, gynecologic and urologic oncologists, radiation therapists, and anesthesiologists.

In addition, a consultant psychiatrist spends 1 day a week at the service and is responsible for, in the following order, caring for staff, families, and patients.

Nursing Staff

The unit staff includes a head nurse, full- and part-time registered nurses, certified nursing assistants, nurse's aides, nursing orderlies, and a unit coordinator (ward clerk). Criteria for nurse selection include: 5 years of broad-based nursing experience, an openness to new ideas and methods, an orientation to people rather than technology, a stable home life with a variety of outside interests, no recent (within 1 year) personal bereavement, and an ability to work as a team member.

The staff-to-patient time ratio has been raised from the hospital level of 5.5 nursing hours per patient to 7.5 hours. This is necessary to assure sufficient staff time to give attention to individual needs of patients and families.

In a controlled cost-analysis study, it was found that the added cost of this nursing time has been more than compensated for by savings due to curtailed irrelevant investigations. Home care nurses' criteria include: the ability to work independently, skills in observing and evaluating physical and emotional symptoms, and experience in community nursing and knowledge of community resources. Consultation nurse criteria include: ability to work independently and to act professionally in a crisis situation, training beyond basic education, teaching experience, and administrative experience.

Volunteers

Palliative Care Service volunteers are people with a wide range of backgrounds, skills, professions, and nationalities. Many have had some experience of loss or death at some point in their lives before coming to the service. In general, volunteers should be at least 25 years of age with that elusive quality of emotional maturity. The best volunteers seem to have a calm and peace about them and are able to communicate this in a quiet and unobtrusive way. They must be flexible in their acceptance of different cultural and religious orientations so that they can serve patients and families without imposing their own values on others. All volunteers are required to attend a training course on the general principles of palliative care as well as an orientation to their duties. They are encouraged to read material about the field and to attend other training courses.

The volunteers work with patients and families in the unit, home care, consultation, and bereavement follow-up programs. They also assist in arranging meetings and social events of the service, in library and office duties, and some in teaching.

Other Clinical Team Members

Other team members include the social worker, chaplain, physiotherapist, dietician, music therapist, and unit coordinator.

The Social Worker. The social worker, with an M.S.W. degree and training in professional counseling, helps patients and families to deal with practical problems of finance, pensions, wills, etc., as well as the broader implications of death and bereavement. The position also includes supervision and evaluation of the bereavement follow-up program, the maintenance of community resource information, and support of other team members.

The Chaplain. A sympathetic chaplain who is a skilled listener and able to meet patients "where they are" rather than where particular religious traditions might suggest they "should be" is a key team member. His presence provides a focus and stimulus for the airing of the metaphysical questions that are invariably present for these patients and their families. The patients' own ministers and other hospital chaplains also participate in ministering to these spiritual needs.

The Physiotherapist. Rather than attempting to improve function, the goal of the palliative care physiotherapist is to help plan activity to maximize the patient's diminishing resources. The physiotherapist is involved in the home care program as well as the unit, and teaches families how to give physiotherapy at home.

The Dietician. The dietician, experienced in the nutritional care of cancer patients, seeks to provide frequent small attractive portions of foods each patient particularly likes. In this phase of the disease, the goal is quality of life rather than improved nutrition.

The Music Therapist. The recent addition to the team of a trained music therapist heralds a 2-year in-depth examination of the potential for music as a catalyst in meeting the needs of patients, families, and staff.

The Unit Coordinator. In other parts of the hospital the unit coordinator or ward clerk orders tests, x-rays, and treatments, as well as maintains ward supplies, etc. As palliative care requires few such tests, the unit coordinator's role has become that of receptionist, information center for patients, families, staff, and others, and assistant in the collection of demographic and evaluation data.

Administrative/Research/Education Staff

The Director. The director as the team leader with the responsibility for the satisfactory operation of the service, spearheads policy development, evaluation, hospital liaison, teaching, and public relations.

The Administrator. The administrator assists the director in details such as ensuring adequate communication and interaction between various components of the service, coordination of research and accumulation of demographic data, procedures and forms design, maintenance of mailing lists, preparation of correspondence and newsletters, administration of palliative care funds and other financial and employment details, and physical arrangements for the unit and offices.

The Education Coordinator. The education coordinator is responsible for coordinating all educational activities, including assistance in organization of training programs, courses, talks, and special functions, supervision of the palliative care library, and arrangement of talks with visitors from outside the hospital and with trainees with the service.

Conclusions and Recommendations

Good medical care, skilled nursing, understanding pastoral care, use of auxiliary services such as physiotherapy, social work, and home care programs, acceptance of help from volunteers and patients' families, attention to the needs of the families—these are the elements of total care that must be developed for providing competent palliative care (4). That the Palliative Care Service has helped patients and families it has served is clear (2, p. 509). Based on our experience, we make some general recommendations:

1. The proportion of palliative care beds in each health care area should be based on the number of cancer deaths in the area (at the Royal Victoria Hospital, the proportion appears to be 4-5 percent of total beds). These beds should be grouped in each institution to form a unit.
2. A home care program should be associated with each unit.
3. The number of nursing personnel on such units should be sufficient to provide approximately 8 nursing hours per patient per day, and the nursing hours should include bereavement follow-up.

4. All medical and paramedical staff should form a multi-disciplinary team, mature volunteers should be included as important members of the team, and the "team approach" should be emphasized.

5. Special training in palliative care should be required for all service staff, including volunteers, in-service education should be a continuing function both within the service and in the institution, and public education should be part of the program objectives.

6. Special attention should be directed to staff stress inherent in this work and to effective staff support.

7. Evaluation should be an on-going priority. Publication of new knowledge, skills, and insights learned through both practical experience and theoretical research will advance the state-of-the-art of palliative care.

References

1. Mount, B. M., Jones, A., & Patterson, A. Death and dying—Attitudes in a teaching hospital. *Urology*, 1974, *4*(8), 741.

2. Mount, B. M. *Report of pilot project (January 1975–January 1977)*. Montreal: Palliative Care Service, Royal Victoria Hospital, 1976.

3. Mount, B. M., Ajemian, I., & Scott, J. F. Use of the Brompton Mixture in treating the chronic pain of malignant disease. *Canadian Medical Association Journal*, 1976, *115*, 122.

4. Shephard, D. A. E. Principles and practice of palliative care. *Canadian Medical Association Journal*, 1976, *116*, 522.

5. Beszterczey, A. Staff stress on a newly developed palliative care service: The psychiatrist's role. *Canadian Psychiatric Association Journal*, 1977, *22*, 347.

Request reprints from Dottie C. Wilson, administrator, Palliative Care Service, Royal Victoria Hospital, 687 Pine Avenue West, Montreal, Quebec, Canada H3A 1A1.

∞∞

HALIFAX (1976)—VICTORIA GENERAL HOSPITAL: A NURSING MODEL

∞∞

NORMA A. WYLIE

School of Nursing, Dalhousie University, and
Department of Nursing, Victoria General Hospital
Halifax, Nova Scotia, Canada

The Hospice Care Program developed from a liaison nursing model in a teaching hospital of Dalhousie University after it appeared that no designated area or full-service personnel would be approved. Highest priority is given to quality nursing and psychosocial care.

Introduction

Living. Dying. What do these words mean? Is there any relationship? Can one have a "good" death? Are we giving quality care to patients who are dying? Are we afraid to care for a dying patient? These and many more questions need to be answered by those of us who care for critically and terminally ill patients and their families and friends. Finding the answers is not an easy task, but I believe for those who truly dare to care for the dying some clues have been discovered, especially during the last decade or so.

There are many problems that seem to contribute to a less than high quality of life for the dying. Since approximately 70 percent of Canadians now die in institutions, it seems appropriate to focus our attention there. Buckingham (1), a medical anthropologist, stated that hospitals, except in the Palliative Care Unit, are poor places for dying:

> There is a tendency to treat the patient as a cancer of the pancreas instead of Bob Buckingham. Doctors and nurses are

trained to diagnose and cure. Dying represents a failure and they fear that, when there is nothing more they can do to cure, there is often nothing more they do. They don't want to get too close. (p. 48)

Taylor (2) describes the drama of death being played in an institution, hospital, or nursing home by many actors (p. 185). She states that the hero may spend much time on stage alone—death has become a lonely process. As the play draws to an end, the physicians appear on stage with decreasing frequency and the nurses bustle on and off, seeming to encourage the hero to play his final scene during the next shift.

Recently a nurse expressed her fears about caring for Mr. J. when he returned to the hospital to die. He had been a patient on her ward several times and the staff had very warm feelings toward him. But, they hoped he would not be admitted to their ward on his final admission. She said, "It would just be too difficult to look after him."

As one deeply concerned about the effectiveness of our health care systems and aware of the potential for improving the lot of the terminally ill, I agreed to share some of my experiences and visions through this article. The focus is on nursing and nurses as they relate to the dying patient. However, I hope it may have meaning to all who read it.

Nurses' Role in Helping the Living to Die

My first real experience with a dying patient began when I was a first-year student nurse

I was on night duty, assigned to work as a float nurse. I was instructed to go to sit with Johnny, a 2-year-old child who was dying. Upon entering the room, I found a curly-headed, blue-eyed boy propped up in the crib under an oxygen tent. Seated on two straight chairs beside him were his parents. I opened the tent, spoke to Johnny, and tried to explain who I was. I also said hello to his parents but they looked so sad and seemed not to want to talk. From 7:00 p.m. until 1:00 a.m. there was very little conversation and no one entered or left the room. I sponged Johnny and tried to make him as comfortable as possible, but I felt so helpless. The silence was almost unbearable as death approached.

About 1:00 a.m. Johnny, with eyes wide open, looked at his parents and said, "Bye-bye, Mommy and Daddy." Life for Johnny had ended. A very frightened student nurse put on the light and presently a stiff, starched night supervisor arrived. She escorted the parents from the room and returned with an intern who pronounced Johnny dead. I was very upset and crying. The supervisor looked at me and said, "Wipe those tears and get busy and bathe this child."

I trust we have progressed some since the above incident occurred, but how much? The work by Quint (3) published 10 years ago was one of the first major studies that related specifically to the role of the nurse and the dying patient. Quint discovered that many nurses are not prepared to cope with the stresses and responsibilities required to care for the dying patient. Her recommendations concerning educational programs that will better prepare both practitioners and teachers have had an influence on present curricula. One may ask what kind of a role model nurses who graduated before 1968 provide in the area of caring for the dying patient.

The attitudinal and behavioral responses toward dying patients characteristic of many nurses today are well documented in the report of a research project carried out by three nurses at the City of Hope Medical Center (4). The report indicates that nurses need further education in order to be aware of their own feelings about death. They need to develop skills that will enable them to deal with dying patients in a realistic and therapeutic manner. The City of Hope team points the way and makes suggestions for more studies: "Effective hospital-based education programs to teach nurses to talk with dying patients are needed now. Studies are needed to test whether education programs effectively change nursing practise" (4, p. 17).

An In-Service Program on Death and Dying

In my search to increase my knowledge and skills in caring for the dying, I attended a 4-week multidisciplinary course at St.

Christopher's Hospice in London. I had followed the writings of
its medical director, Dr. Cicely Saunders, from the late 1950s
until the present. Her articles published in 1959 and reprinted in
1976 (5) have given inspiration and help to many. She states:
"The answer to suffering lies not in legislation, but in education—education of doctors, nurses and of the general public" (5,
p. 3). What I learned during my time at St. Christopher's was
invaluable in helping me with the work discussed in this article.

In 1974 I directed a research project that was undertaken on
a surgical ward at The Victoria General Hospital in Halifax,
Nova Scotia. Six months after its commencement, it was extended to a medical ward. One independent variable of the study
was an in-service program based on nurses' identified needs. In a
study for her doctoral dissertation, Price (6) clearly stated that
an in-service program should be based upon the nurses' concep-
tion of their personal needs. The surgical ward in the study had
a large number of terminal cancer patients. Therefore, it was not
surprising that the assessment of the nurses' needs gave priority
to assistance in the management of dying patients and the
support of their families. The assessment of the nurses' needs on
the medical ward later showed a similar need. It was then
decided that a program should be planned to try to meet some
of these needs.

In planning the program, nurses' needs were based on the
needs of the dying patient, which are physiological, psychosocial, and spiritual. The next question to be addressed was how
to plan the program. Quint (7) and others identified problems of
communication that nurses experience, particularly when trying
to talk with patients who have a life-threatening illness or who
are dying. A common question asked by many nurses is, "What
do I say when a patient unexpectedly asks, 'Am I going to
die?' " We recognized there is no easy answer, but in discussion
with the head nurse of the study ward it seemed educationally
sound to plan some group experience. We agreed that the
physiological needs were being met fairly well and we should
concentrate on the psychosocial and spiritual needs. To assist us
with the program, I felt we needed the presence of a chaplain.
The role of the hospital chaplain does not seem to be clearly
understood by many care givers, especially as it relates to care

of the dying patient. They assume that chaplains function only in the traditional role of being called at the "end" to administer the Sacrament, say a prayer, or perform other appropriate religious ceremonies. However, many theological institutes now provide clinical pastoral education programs with special experiences related to the dying patient (8, 9, pp. 37–43). Therefore, it seemed appropriate to invite a chaplain to share with me the leadership for a group experience.

The plan for an in-service program was developed in collaboration with the head nurse, the chaplain, and myself. We developed the following objectives:

1. To help us become more aware of our own feelings and attitudes in facing the reality of death.
2. To increase our communication skills in caring for dying persons and their families.

It was acknowledged that to begin to devleop a sense of self-awareness, bring about attitudinal change, and develop some interpersonal skills would take time and all we could do was open some doors. To provide some opportunity for all the nurses who wished to participate and work within the constraints of staffing patterns, we decided to plan five $1\frac{1}{2}$ hour small group sessions in close sequence. We felt it was important to have a commitment from all participants, which included attendance at all sessions unless ill. The head nurse was able to allow only a small number of nursing staff off the ward, but many came in on their off-duty time so that most groups contained five or six nurses. We also agreed to have interdisciplinary groups with a maximum size of 12 members, including the two leaders. The head nurse accepted the responsibility for inviting members of other health professions to participate.

The first series was truly interdisciplinary, with eight nurses—including the head nurse, five staff nurses, one nursing assistant, and myself—the chaplain, a social worker, a dietitian, and the hospital librarian in attendance. At the first session objectives were discussed with participants and a contract established. Group discussion was fostered in various ways using patient care situations whenever possible. Use of role-playing techniques was helpful in trying to identify one's own feelings and in developing some communication skills. Indeed, the technique we used was supported by Barton and Crowder (10), who, in describing a course they developed at Vanderhill University Medical Center, stated: "We have found role playing to be a particularly useful instructional aid in teaching in the area, especially in the instruction of multidisciplinary student groups" (p. 244). To complement the group experience, participants were given one or two articles to read that related to specific issues raised during the session.

An evaluation was done not only after each session but also at the conclusion of the first series. Minor changes were made but the same format and processes were used for the second and succeeding series. The five sessions were repeated until all nurses from the ward under study had attended. Because of some staff changes, it was necessary to repeat the series eight times. Although this committed us to considerable time, the chaplain and I considered it to be well worthwhile. The chaplain wrote the following in an evaluation:

> This was the first time I have been involved in a consultative process. I feel the fact of contracting for a set number of sessions and having a commitment from participants in terms of time and attendance helped facilitate participation, especially in the area of group solidarity and individual sharing of personal feelings related to one's own eventual death, feelings of grief, and feelings related to caring for dying persons.

Upon completion of the sessions, the nurses were given a questionnaire as a means of evaluating the in-service program. We followed the one developed by Popoff (11), which is a 36-item tool with ranked options that range from two to seven categories. In this tool high scores indicate more favorable attitudes toward death and dying and also the ability to care satisfactorily for the dying patient in terms of his psychosocial skills. Because attitudes were measured only at the conclusion of the in-service program, there was no initial measurement from which to compute changes in attitudes or ability. A control group of nurses from a comparable ward, but not exposed to the program, was given the questionnaire to provide a comparative analysis.

It was hypothesized that nurses who participated in the planned in-service program have more favorable attitudes toward death and dying than those who did not participate. There were 22 in each group. The analysis proved the hypothesis to be correct, which was very encouraging. The results supported the belief that an in-service program, based on identified needs of the learner, could affect change. Although the tool was not designed to measure nursing practice per se, it seems reasonable to assume that the findings should have some effect on quality of care given by those who participated in the group experience.

Design for a Nursing Model

The impact of the group sessions was far-reaching. Nurses in other parts of the hospital expressed a desire for a similar experience, as did a number of personnel from other disciplines. Physicians were the exceptions. Although attempts were made to include them in each session, we did not have much success. A review of some studies may help us understand physician reluctance to participate. A study by Herman Feifel (12) comparing members of different professional groups determined that medical students and physicians tend to be people who are afraid of death and that physicians fear death more than do members of other professional groups. Mount (13) reported similar attitudes and behaviors from findings of a questionnaire circulated to different staff members of the Royal Victoria Hospital in Montreal. He stated:

> Isolation, suspicion and distrust develop owing to the lack of communication between patients, family members, nurses and physicians. This is fostered by physicians' reluctance to inform the patient of the diagnosis and prognosis, a natural preference to treat disease rather than to deal with personal and social problems, and an endemic denial of death. (p. 119)

The request for help by many staff members and the problems associated with caring for terminally ill patients and their families by all care givers could not be ignored. A proposal, based on the model of the Palliative Care Unit in Montreal, was prepared by the associate director of nursing service and myself. It was presented to the administrative and senior medical staff of The Victoria General Hospital and accepted in principle. A working party committee, called the Hospice Care Committee, was established to develop a detailed program for the establishment of a Palliative Care Unit. The following disciplines were represented on the committee: nursing (service and education), medicine (two family physicians, a psychiatrist, and an internist), social work, and chaplaincy.

Our early deliberations were influenced by the example set at St. Christopher's Hospice and the work of Dr. Cicely Saunders—herself a nurse. In an article written in 1976 (14), she stated, "Terminal care demands a professionalism of a very high degree on the part of those who are writing the prescription for care—a professionalism which involves nurses, doctors and social workers who must involve and discuss the care with the patients and their relatives" (p. 3). The concepts on which St. Christopher's was built and functions today formed the basis for our preliminary planning at The Victoria General Hospital. They are:

1. Dying with dignity.
2. The patient does not die alone and abandoned.
3. Pain is controlled.
4. The patient's family is involved in the care.
5. A bereavement service provides assistance to families.
6. Psychiatric participation.

Several meetings were held to develop our own philosophy and objectives. We subscribed to the belief that the word *hospice* symbolizes physical, psychological, and spiritual care toward a quality of life that should give meaning to living and dying. We also focused on the total community, i.e., ambulatory, hospital, and/or home care and all those involved. This included the patient, family, and the care givers including the volunteer. A staff nurse on the committee wrote the following philosophy based on our beliefs:

PHILOSOPHY OF HOSPICE PROGRAM

To provide a dying person with comfort, love, and peace,
An atmosphere of easiness to help those feeling weak,

To show concern, to listen well, to those who still have much to tell,
With smiling faces and physical touch,
We can bring each person so very much.
For the sickness they have requires loving attention,
Medical procedures need little mention.

It is too for those left behind
That our work must be kind,
Tempered with love and forged with care,
The burden of absence is brought to bear.
Help is provided to those in the fight
To view death in a more positive light.
The lonely and disheartened look to you
With eyes questioning "Is it really true?"

A private area that surrounds one with friends
And unhappiness, our work attempts to mend.
To let the family have a share
Giving them purpose for being there.

For once this purpose is carried through
Many dear faces won't be so blue.
They'll have in their hearts contentment and peace
Due to the works within the hospice.

Yvonne Hennebury, R.N.
July 1976

It was a simple task to develop our overall and specific objectives once we accepted such a philosophy.

Objectives

Our overall objective was to encourage a more positive and constructive effort in discovering ways in which our real concern for the dying person and the family can be expressed to them during the dying and grieving process. Specific objectives were to:

1. Provide successful management of pain and suffering.
2. Provide a cheerful environment, which will assist the person to live with dignity while dying.
3. Permit the person and the family their right to become involved in their plan of care.
4. Help survivors in the grieving process.

5. Blend the skills of the nurses, doctors, clergy, social workers, volunteers, and others who wish to become involved in the care of the dying person.
6. Demonstrate to learners and others a special approach in the care of the dying person and the family.
7. Support both the person who wishes to die at home, and the family.

Although our original proposal was programmed for a Hospice Unit, it became apparent after several meetings and discussions with a number of medical and administrative staff the present circumstances prevented the establishment of a hospice. Also, we were beginning to explore alternative ways of implementing the hospice philosophy and questioning the need for attitudinal changes toward care of the dying versus environmental changes. Is it possible to improve quality of care without a special unit?

It was indeed fortuitous that about this time three of us from the Hospice Care Committee had the opportunity to attend the first International Seminar on Terminal Care in Montreal. We had the rare privilege of listening to and talking and sharing with many people who had a genuine common concern—caring for the dying. Among the guest speakers was Dr. Cicely Saunders, who spent a day in Halifax after the seminar. She met with members of our committee, at which time we explored with her the possibility of developing a proposal for a Hospice Care Program. This was heartily endorsed by her.

The next task of the committee was to compare a Hospice Unit and a Hospice Care Program. A visit to the Palliative Care Unit in Montreal provided some of us with some up-to-date information on this model. We also had available to us a brochure on a Hospice Care Program that had been in operation at St. Luke's Hospital in New York for approximately 2 years (15). There, they formed a multidisciplinary Symptom Control Team with a twofold purpose: "primarily, to focus on the real needs of the cancer patient and those close to him in order to enable them to maintain the fullest possible life, and secondly, to educate the medical community in alternate methods of caring for these patients" (15, p. 1).

Some of the major aspects of each model that we identified appear in the following table.

Hospice (Palliative Care) Unit	Hospice Care Program
Legislation would be needed to establish this.	This could be more easily formed and the idea of hospice care established through inspiration.
Would provide for continuity of care. Control of care easier here.	Would provide for a much wider educational/in-service program. May reach larger numbers of persons.
Fewer people and time to "sell" philosophy and to effect change.	Would provide for probable education of both medical and nursing students.
Would need a medical director and support from medical staff, i.e., pain control and dying with dignity.	Family physician and others (e.g., those "outside" of hospital structure) could more easily be included.
	Could start immediately to meet some of the staff needs related to the dying patient and his family.
	Consultative services could cover a wider area.

It is self-evident that both of these models, the Palliative Care Unit and the Hospice Care Program, patterned after the philosophy and design of St. Christopher's Hospice, are providing a special service to the care of terminally ill patients and their families. However, in the words of the founder of the hospice movement, "We must keep on welcoming, sharing and testing new ideas" (14, p. 1). And so we looked again at some of the expressed needs of the staff and patients at The Victoria General Hospital and the community it serves. The group who had declared most vocally the need for assistance related to death and dying was the nursing staff. Therefore, the design for a nursing model already had a beginning with the in-service program on the two study wards. There was a need now to expand it and to develop a more formal structure based on the philosophy and concepts of St. Christopher's Hospice.

Why should there be a nursing model? There appears to be significant literature and research indicating a need to improve the quality and kind of care that is presently being given to terminally ill patients. To achieve this objective would require the development of new leadership patterns of nurses caring for these patients. Since nurses make up the largest groups of care givers, a unique opportunity is provided to initiate, together with other health professionals, carefully planned care. Quint (16) challenges us with the following statement: "Any nurse who is truly concerned about personalizing patient care through her own efforts must reckon with the reality that to do so means a willingness to 'rock the boat' of the health care system as it presently functions" (p. 267).

One staff nurse (17), who dares to care for the dying, has this to say:

> We expend so much energy running from it. Remember how frightened you were to give that first injection? The fear lessened after you learned the principles and had some experiences. It's the same with death and dying—the more knowledgeable and experienced you become about it, the less frightening it appears. In giving to the dying, the living find reward. (17, p. 89)

What this staff nurse, and others like her, is saying and doing does not necessarily require a special building or unit in which to give the care that the dying need. What then is required? To assist us in trying to answer this vital question, a conceptual framework (Figure 1) was developed. This became our road map in designing a nursing model. This framework is based on our belief that to provide quality of life to the dying, we should acknowledge living from birth until death. Paul Tournier describes it (18) as "a man in movement, continually undergoing change, a man living a history, unfolding from his birth until his death. The very movement implies meaning in life."

The framework is designed by identifying certain processes that need to be understood before we can begin to develop a nursing care plan. The process that encapsulates all others is called the *living process*. What does this mean to you? One patient, who was dying, said to a student nurse, "I'm only half a man now." Glen Davidson (19) has given much insight and guidance to those of us who work with dying persons and their families. He believes that in order to try to understand what

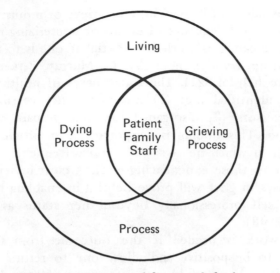

FIGURE 1 Conceptual framework for hospice program.

dying means to us we must first consider what our expectations for living are: "For some of us, dying means the experience of discovering who we really are. Then 'dying' becomes the most revelatory event of our life" (p. 26).

The *dying process* is embodied within the framework. Dying is as much a psychosocial and spiritual reality as a biological one. Therefore, an awareness of the dynamics involved is essential if we are going to give more than physical care. Three physicians (20) have this to say in an article addressed to an understanding of the dying process: "Medical achievement has created a need for better understanding of and response to the dying process" (p. 62).

The final process that is identified in the framework is the *grieving process*. Figure 1 demonstrates diagrammatically the interlocking of each process and the interrelationships of one on the other. The convergence of the processes in the center shows that at certain times the dying person, the family, and the care givers may be having similar experiences. At this juncture, as well as moving through the phases back to the periphery, we need to understand the dynamics of each process. Although grief and grieving are normal responses to the loss of a loved one,

many of us have not learned how to grieve or mourn effectively.
Knowledge of the sequence of events characterizing normal grief
and of the meaning of each is essential if one is to help wisely.
Findings from research done by C. Murray Parkes and John
Bowlby are helpful (21). The four phases of healthy mourning
that they identified are: (1) numbness, (2) yearning for the
deceased person, (3) disorganization and despair, and (4) re-
organization. This finding is supported in an article written by
Engel (22), in which he says: "The nurse frequently is called on
to minister to those experiencing grief. A clear understanding of
the processes in grief will prove helpful in enabling the nurse to
extend herself professionally beyond her status as a humane
person" (p. 98).

Grief work is needed if the outcome from the grieving
process is to be positive and allow one to return to healthy,
normal living. Do nurses have the necessary skills and knowledge
to become involved in this special work? The whole area of
bereavement is a topic within itself. However, a discussion of the
grieving process is not complete without a brief reference to
bereavement. Parkes and others have documented the effects of
bereavement on physical and mental illness, and thus in developing our nursing model we have been cognizant of the role nurses
should and can play. This is well supported in an article by Joy
Rogers and Mary Vachon (23) in which they too believe nurses
can help the bereaved: "By virtue of their personal caring roles
and their positions within institutions and in the community at
large, nurses are uniquely suited to carry more responsibility in
providing service to the bereaved" (p. 1).

Figure 1 helped us to identify the processes that need to be
understood. A brief description of these seemed to indicate that
our conceptual framework was incomplete unless it identified
the needs of all involved. Only then could we begin to plan a
learning process that would change some of the present beliefs
and practices relating to death and dying. Charlotte Epstein (24)
says:

> The dying process has been observed and recorded; the behavior of
> nurses and other medical personnel has been described; and the
> responses of bereaved families have become a part of the contem-
> porary data that help to fill the gap in our knowledge about

dying. However, it simply is not fair to the care-givers or the dying patient to expect their interaction to begin with only a background of required reading. (p. 3)

The information in the literature needs to be made operational.

The needs of all persons involved in the processes just described were categorized into three major headings, as care, education, and assistance. These are diagrammed in Table 1.

Nurses are the primary care givers for whom this model has been designed. However, it is not the intent of the author, who basically designed this model, or the members who improved and endorsed it to exclude anyone. The care of the dying is not an individual work, but one that is shared—shared with relatives, all members of the health care team, and, as much as possible, the patient. The interdisciplinary membership of the Hospice Care Committee speaks for itself. Without each other one can do

TABLE 1

Needs	Patient	Family	Care Givers
Care	Physical Institution Psycho- a. Clinic social b. In-patient Spiritual Home	Assist with patient care Supportive a. Psychosocial b. Spiritual	All staff members and volunteers Supportive (from others)
Education	Knowledge regarding own illness a. Diagnosis b. Prognosis c. Treatment Knowledge regarding processes in Figure 1 Living Dying Grieving	Same as listed for patient and bereaving	Same as patient/family *How* to meet self and patient/family needs Trained minds Trained hands Educated hearts
Assistance	Benefit from other doctor's advice How to help care givers, other patients	Involve in short/long term plan of care	Maximize each other's resources

very little. However, it is my firm conviction that to meet the majority of the needs identified in Table 1, nurses can and are providing care leadership.

One of the limitations of this nursing model is in the area of pain control. As nurses, we cannot prescribe pain "killers." However, studies relating to pain control indicate that nurses could do much better if their knowledge and skills were increased. McCaffery (25) says: "Doctors may underprescribe and nurses may not give what is needed—and patients may suffer unnecessarily" (p. 1586). In an earlier article (26) she states: "It seems that in many instances how well the patient is able to handle his pain is dependent on what his nurse does" (p. 1227). Physical pain is only one aspect to consider.

What about emotional and spiritual pain? Patients need help and understanding in trying to cope with these painful distresses. Modern medicine has done much to alleviate many forms of pain, but often suffering remains even when pain is relieved. Cicely Saunders (14) says: "Much can be done by calm, dependable nursing but it is the real listener who helps most of all. The nurse often has the greatest opportunity to fill this role and can therefore give her patient his greatest solace. Suffering is intolerable only when nobody cares" (p. 18). Each faith has its own understanding and belief of what it means to suffer. The Apostle Paul, in his teachings to the early Christians, said, "for when I am weak, then am I strong" (Corinthians 12:10 KJV).

The design of this nursing model for a Hospice Care Program is an attempt to explore yet another approach to improve the quality of care of the dying person. The conceptual framework is presented as a blueprint to help nurses identify their learning needs. The results of the findings from the questionnaire related to death and dying showed that learning did take place with the in-service program that was based on the identified needs of the learner. It therefore appears there is a shared responsibility between the institution and each nurse to plan and participate in an appropriate program.

The institution that is committed to quality of care for the terminally ill may wish to consider the employment of at least one nurse who has special preparation and skills in the field of thanatology. Nurses find this field a rich, rewarding experience.

They not only give total patient care on a selected basis, but also teach hospital personnel how to develop or improve their interactions with the dying person. One nurse specialist (27) says,

> Working with dying patients can be a tremendously growing experience if the nurse primarily responsible for the patient's care is provided a mechanism whereby she, too, may go through a grieving process. It is this nurse grieving process that I believe is the key to enabling a nurse to keep giving to dying patients. (p. 1490)

It is not expected that all nurses should or could become specialists in caring for the dying person. But I believe each nurse has a responsibility to develop personal self-awareness and to acquire a repertory of behaviors that will be helpful in the nurse/patient interaction, be those situations physical, psychosocial, or spiritual. It does not necessarily require a special edifice like a hospice or a palliative care unit to do this. What better edifice can anyone build than a therapeutic use of self? An affirmation from a nurse (17) who does care says: "Caring is risky but you don't lose by giving of yourself. If you dare to become so involved with a dying person that you even cry, don't be afraid. Perhaps some day someone will cry at your passing" (p. 90).

I trust the journey throughout this article has been worthwhile for those who have taken it with me. Mine began with the 2-year-old, blue-eyed boy and has had many detours along the way. I am grateful for the inspiration and help I have received from many committed to providing dignity and quality of life to the dying. I have been able to acknowledge only a few. To Dr. Cicely Saunders I owe a special thanks of gratitude for steering my journey toward the hospice movement. St. Christopher's has opened many doors and provided a model of caring for all to emulate. It has given us a gift, which is a new professional attitude toward dying and death, with the realization and conscious acceptance of dying and death as part of being born and part of the struggle of life. "For none of us liveth to himself, and no man dieth to himself" (Romans 14:7 KJV).

References

1. Diebel, L. The man who "died" to prove a point: hospitals are poor places for dying. *MacLean's,* January 1977, 48.
2. Taylor, C. *In horizontal orbit.* New York: Holt, 1970.
3. Quint, J. C. *The nurse and the dying patient.* New York: Macmillan, 1967.
4. Padilla, G., Baker, V., & Dolan, V. *Interacting with dying patients.* Duarte, Calif.: City of Hope National Medical Centre, 1975.
5. Saunders, C. Care of the dying (a series of articles). *Nursing Times,* 1976, *72*(26).
6. Price, E. *Learning needs of registered nurses.* New York: Columbia Teachers College Press, 1967.
7. Benoliel, Quint, J. Talking to patients about death. *Nursing Forum,* 1970, *9*(3), 255–269.
8. Cavanaugh, J. The chaplain and the dying patient. *Hospital Progress,* November 1971, 35–40.
9. Nighswonger, C. Ministry to the dying as a learning encounter. In D. Bane & A. H. Kutcher (Eds.), *Death and ministry: Pastoral care of the dying and bereaved.* New York: Seabury, 1975.
10. Barton, D., & Crowder, M. The use of role playing techniques as an instructional aid in teaching about dying, death and bereavement. *Omega,* 1975, *6*(3), 243–250.
11. Popoff, D. Death and dying—how do you really feel about it? *Nursing '74,* 1974, *4*(11), 58–63.
12. Feifel, H. Is death's sting sharper for the doctor? *Medical World News,* October 1967, 77.
13. Mount, B. M. The problem of caring for the dying in a general hospital; the palliative care unit as a possible solution. *C.M.A. Journal,* 1976, *115*, 97–98, 119–130, 179–185.
14. Saunders, C. The hospice movement. *Nursing Times,* 1976, *72*(26).
15. St. Luke's Hospital Center, New York, *Hospice pilot project,* 1975.
16. Benoliel, Quint, J. Death. *Nursing Forum,* 1970, *9*(3), 255–267.
17. Ufema, J. Dare to care for the dying. *American Journal of Nursing,* 1976, *76*(1), 88–90.
18. Tournier, P. *The seasons of life.* Richmond, Va.: John Knox, 1961.
19. Davidson, G. *Living with dying.* Minneapolis, Augsburg, 1975.
20. Tomm, K., Williams, J., & Matheson, G. Understanding the dying process. *Canadian Family Physician,* 1976, *22*, 62–65.
21. Parkes, M. Seeking and finding a lost object. *Social Science and Medicine,* 1970, *4*, 187–201.
22. Engel, G. Grief and grieving. *American Journal of Nursing,* 1964, *64*(9), 93–98.
23. Rogers, J., & Vachon, M. Nurses can help the bereaved. *The Canadian Nurse,* 1975, *71*(6), 1–4.

24. Epstein, C. *Nursing the dying patient.* Reston, Va.: Reston, 1975.
25. McCaffery, M. Undertreatment of acute pain with narcotics. *The American Journal of Nursing,* October 1976, 1586–1591.
26. McCaffery, M. Nursing intervention for bodily pain. *The American Journal of Nursing,* June 1976, 1224–1227.
27. Songstegard, L., et al. The grieving nurse. *The American Journal of Nursing,* September 1976, 1490–1492.

NEW HAVEN (1974)—CHARACTERISTICS OF
A HOSPICE PROGRAM OF CARE

SYLVIA A. LACK

Hospice, Inc., New Haven, Connecticut

Under physician leadership, Hospice, Inc., started a home care program for terminally ill cancer patients and their families in March 1974. This paper is based on the 3-year evaluation by the medical director who argues that priority of care should be directed to physical needs, managed in a problem-oriented approach.

Introduction

Hospice, Inc., has just completed a 3-year contract with the National Cancer Institute. The goal was to demonstrate continuing care at home for patients whose prognosis precludes an aggressive rehabilitative endeavor. We wanted to find out if this mode of management was acceptable to the American public— patients, family, professionals, and the general community.

The National Cancer Institute contract enabled Hospice to develop a demonstration project free from the usual financial and bureaucratic constraints. We were able to focus on the needs of patients and their families and develop a creative program designed to meet these needs. There was concern at the outset that palliative home care would be unacceptable in this country. I was frequently told that "Americans are hospital oriented; when Americans are sick they want to be in the hospital." "Nobody dies at home in this country. The society is not set up for it." "We don't have a stiff upper lip over here, you know. We never give up." "Palliative care is against the American way of life."

Despite all these gloomy prophesies, Hospice has demonstrated that home care is very much desired by a proportion of the population. Families are prepared to accept great hardship to keep a loved one home, and at the appropriate time intensive personal care or palliative care is welcomed. Furthermore, a service emphasizing quality of life rather than diagnosis and cure can be integrated into professional and lay concepts of health care. We have also shown through the evaluation study that this service benefits patients and families alike and that these benefits are measurable. This achievement has not come easily; many mistakes were made along the way, and grappling with innovation caused inevitable inefficiencies in use of staff time. Out of our painful experience have evolved program characteristics we believe are essential to the delivery of effective hospice care to the terminally ill and their families. They are (1):

1. Coordinated home care—inpatient beds under a central autonomous hospice administration.
2. Skilled symptom control (physical, sociological, psychological, and spiritual).
3. Physician directed services.
4. Provision of care by an interdisciplinary *team*.
5. Services available on a 24-hour-a-day, 7-day-a-week, on-call basis with emphasis on availability of medical and nursing skills.
6. Patient/family regarded as the unit of care.
7. Bereavement follow-up.
8. Use of volunteers as an integral part of the interdisciplinary team.
9. Structured staff support and communication systems.
10. Patients should be accepted to the program on the basis of health needs, not ability to pay.

Home Care—Inpatient Facilities

Hospice began life in a very different fashion than any then existing hospice. We started home care without any backup beds and have continued thus for over 3 years. This was a painless, nonthreatening method of introducing the concept to the health care community, as few of them operate in the home. Visiting nurse associations' involvement in planning the program and their willingness to share the care in many homes was crucial to providing optimum terminal care. Another benefit was that we expanded our concepts of what was possible at home. During the study period over 65 percent of patients died at home— much above the national average. Never were we in any controversy with established medical opinion about the appropriateness of such deaths despite such radical departure from the usual locale of care. Our experience also bore out the original contention that these patients require an intensity of care not usually provided by nursing homes. Out of the 34.3 percent who did not die at home, only 3.4 percent died in nursing homes.

There were various disadvantages. We saw many patients adamantly refuse to go into a facility, usually because they had experienced, on previous admissions, a deficiency in the type of intensive personal care they needed. Several of these died at home with symptoms that could have been controlled in a hospice bed. Other home deaths threw a very great strain on the family. It was painful to watch the symptomatic deterioration of many patients as continuity of care was lost on hospital admission. Techniques of comfort that had worked well in the home were ignored by a system geared to investigation, diagnosis, and cure—but not to comfort care. The past 3 years of experience indicates that the optimum hospice care can only be delivered when home care and inpatient beds are under the same central, autonomous hospice administration.

In North America there have been several innovative approaches to the provisions of these two components. Hospice is following the St. Christopher's model of building a 44-bed hospital to provide a therapeutic environment uniquely qualified to back up the home care program. At the Royal Victoria Hospital in Montreal, Dr. Balfour Mount has created a 14-bed Palliative Care Unit within an acute general hospital. The unit functions largely as a separate entity, with its own philosophy of care and its own relaxation of hospital regulations. St. Luke's Hospital in New York has taken yet another approach. It provides an interdisciplinary hospice team that attends patients with a terminal illness in the hospital wherever they may be located. Special provisions are made for hospice patients in terms of family visiting, children visiting, hair washing, and the like. The team works closely with the ward staff to provide the best care for the patient and follows the patient and family in the home setting.

Symptom Control

There is far too much talk in death and dying circles in this country about psychological and emotional problems, and far too little about making the patient comfortable. Any group concerned with service to the dying should be talking about smoothing sheets, rubbing bottoms, relieving constipation, and sitting up at night. Counseling a person who is lying in a wet bed is ludicrous. Discomfort looms large in the lives of patients with a terminal illness and must be of importance to physicians if they are to treat the whole person. A certain amount of interdisciplinary role blurring may be necessary to ensure patient comfort at all times.

If people are cared for with common sense and basic professional skills, with detailed attention to self-evident problems and physical needs, then patients and families themselves cope with many of their emotional crises. Without pain, well nursed, with bowels controlled, clean mouths, and a caring friend available, psychological problems fall into manageable perspective.

Any physician who is dealing with a number of terminally ill patients must become interested in symptom control and skilled in the management of the various types of physical distress caused by an incurable illness. Sadly, the terminal stage has been defined by some as beginning at the moment when the doctor says, "there is nothing more to be done," and then begins to withdraw subtly from the patient. Patients, of course, are very well aware when this happens. There is never a time when "nothing more can be done." There may indeed be nothing more that can be done to cure the disease, but there are always further measures to be taken for the comfort of the patient and the well-being of the family.

Severe cancer pain can be controlled by narcotics and adjuvant drugs. The narcotic should be titrated to the patient's need and used regularly to maintain pain control. Taken in regular oral doses, a narcotic can be used for many months without a need to escalate the dose. Hospice has demonstrated the regular narcotic use is accepted by doctors and patients and that oral morphine is a good substitute for oral heroin. In fact in May 1977, St. Christopher's in London changed from oral heroin to oral morphine (2).

Every physician should have a virtually inexhaustable store of remedies for all the common problems that we meet in terminal disease. We have found it useful to take a problem-oriented approach, treating each symptom almost as a disease in itself to be diagnosed and treated. Thus the patient becomes not Mr. A. with incurable cancer, but Mr. A., the man with the severe pain for which we can do a great deal. This enables the team to approach the patient with a positive, optimistic, realistic attitude. The effect of such an approach on the patient and family may be dramatic.

Physician Directed Services

Patients with a terminal illness and their families consistently report their feelings of medical abandonment. One of our new patients said sadly, "I feel as though I have lost Dr. Q. somewhere along the way." It is often the loss of their doctor's interest that patients fear the most. Patients who elect to remain at home for their last weeks may find themselves cut off from effective medical care because many physicians do not make home visits. We see patients seriously ill, suffering from vomiting, pain, and other controllable symptoms, bedfast at home, who have not seen a doctor for many weeks. Others find that, if they do struggle to the office or to a hospital clinic, they frequently see a resident, while the person they regard as their doctor is seeing patients who can be cured. It is vital to the psychological and physical well-being of the patient with terminal illness that the physician is a key figure in the care received.

Medical direction of the program was also vital in gaining

acceptance by the medical community. Initially physicians feared that once referred to the hospice program, patients would be on a "one-way escalator to death" regardless of improvements in their condition or new disease treatment advances. We demonstrated that competent medical overview identified misdiagnoses, remissions, complications amenable to hospital treatment, and patients referred too early in the course of their disease.

Provision of Care by an Interdisciplinary Team

The management of the dying must be a team concern. The team includes the dying patient and immediate family, doctor, chaplain, nurses, social worker, volunteers, secretaries, and other health care personnel. Continuity of management forms an important part of the total care. Interdisciplinary care must not be synonymous with fragmented care in which the bewildered patient does not know who is in charge or who is dealing with which problem. Real teamwork mandates that the interdisciplinary staff sit down together at regular conferences to work out a plan of care for the patient/family and to learn each other's languages.

Real teamwork includes the support and supply staff, without whom the front liners would collapse. On the first home visit the team concept is always clearly explained and a handwritten list of the team personnel placed by the phone. Recently, on reading the list, a wife exclaimed, "But what about Kay and Jill (our secretaries)? They are the only ones who've helped me so far." We have learned that it is only by constant listening to the patient/family that we can even approach an understanding of the basic truths of good, relevant caring.

An attitude of openness and cooperation and the philosophy of an extended team maintains good working relationships with other essential personnel. Hospice seeks to complement, not duplicate, the services tendered by others. There is no room in terminal care for interagency rivalries or interdisciplinary turf guards. Two examples of the extended team in New Haven are the visting nurse associations and the community pharmacists. One of the latter made Dilaudid suppositories from cocoa butter on a weekend after 17 phone calls had failed to locate any. Imaginative individuals prepared to go to extraordinary lengths for a person in pain help make Hospice work.

Service Availability on a 24-Hour Basis

A husband who reluctantly placed his wife in a convalescent home for the last 3 months of her life described the kind of stress that forced her admission. He remembered, with vivid horror, the time her gastrostomy tube fell out at 3:00 a.m. and he tried to replace it according to phone instructions from an unknown emergency room physician.

Such emergencies all too often occur at night and weekends when help is scarce. The fear and anxiety engendered by even the thought of such crises causes many families to give up home care. Provision of emergency availability of medical and nursing staff gives families and patients the security and support they need to continue.

The experience of the families regarding available help must tally with what they are told. "You're very difficult to get hold of," insisted one daughter. She was trying in vain to tell her mother's physician that, prior to the present admission, she had tried to reach him for 3 days because her mother had severe vaginal bleeding. Finally, a dash to the emergency room resulted in immediate admission. No amount of firm reassurance by the doctor, as he tried to persuade her to take mother home again, could blot out the fear and anxiety of those 3 days. We sometimes find that families test out our 24-hour availability and call us out for some trivial (to us) reason. Once they discover we are really there, they stop testing and do not abuse the service.

Patient and Family Regarded as the Unit of Care

Objective support for this concept now comes from the evaluation study (3) that indicates that the family member primarily carrying the burden of care suffers more anxiety, depression, and social malfunctioning than the patients themselves. This finding applied to both hospice and nonhospice groups.

"Nothing that we do should serve to separate someone who is dying from his family. There may be moments of difficulty or even despair, but it is of paramount importance that they come through to the end together. The journey itself may ease the next stages for those who have to go on living afterwards," says Dr. Saunders. A terminal illness is not like an acute illness. In an acute illness, although the short-term stress may be great, the long-term hope and anticipation is that full family function will be restored. In a terminal illness every member of the family is pulled in and affected by the illness. Adjustments to living without the patient begin before death, as functions previously fulfilled by the patient have to be taken over by other members of the family. We must aim to involve the family from the beginning.

Upon admission to an inpatient facility, the family who has been nursing the patient at home has invaluable experience and advice to offer the professionals on the precise details of care. These include what is the most comfortable position, how frequently medication needs to be given to keep the pain under control, and certain expressions unique to this particular patient. For example, a 19-year-old was labeled confused and then heavily sedated after he had repeatedly cried out in a terrified fashion that a big red engine was in the room. It was only after his death that the family told how it was the fire service who brought his oxygen to the home when he had breathing difficulties. He was trying to communicate to the hospital staff a need for oxygen and help in breathing. He was not asking to be sedated.

Time is well spent when we listen sympathetically to a husband telling of his fears for his own health because he has been passing blood in his urine for 2 months. Many family members deny their own needs because of the demands of looking after the sick person. Their own needs still exist, however, and they worry about them. Eventually they feel neglected and may resent the patient for drawing attention away from themselves.

Over and over again we hear our families say, "We could not

have done it without you." One daughter told us that the Hospice staff were her "backbone." "You held me up so that my hands were free to care for my father," she said. Families can manage for a much longer period of time if they have professional support immediately available to them.

Bereavement Follow-up

A hospice program provides emotional support for surviving families during bereavement. Care does not stop with death of the patient. We consider bereavement follow-up to be preventive health care and, through trial and error, have evolved a unique program combining early follow-up by the primary nurse and long term follow-up by volunteers. We continue to visit the family on a scheduled or emergency basis right through death and on into the mourning period. Families require assistance as they endure suffering caused by the separation. In the first year after bereavement, there is increased vulnerability to illness, which is reflected in a 40 percent increase in the mortality rate of widowers. Other consequences include increased alcoholism, reactive depression, and long term detrimental effects to children caused by loss of a parent. Dr. Colin Murray Parkes (4) believes that simple friendly visiting to give the survivors an opportunity to express their grief and discuss the terminal illness and death can go a long way toward mitigating the ill effects of bereavement. In our program the first bereavement visits are made by the primary nurse who was involved with the care of the patient before death. This gives the family an opportunity to discuss questions such as "Should we have kept him at home? Should we have taken him to the hospital? Was it worth continuing with that unpleasant treatment for so long? Should we have pressed her to continue with chemotherapy? Why didn't she go to the doctor as soon as she felt the lump?" Many of these questions can easily be cleared up by frank and open discussion. Left unattended, they grow and fester in the minds of the bereaved to cause much unnecessary suffering. Subsequent visits are made by trained volunteers.

Volunteers—Used as an Integral Part of
the Home Care Team

"You medical folk are all very nice," said one husband, "but the
real people are better." He was referring to our volunteers. Lay
volunteers can be used to help the family with the day-to-day
tasks of running a household. The family member may be pulled
away from these tasks by the demands of caring for the patient,
and it is the volunteer who can provide help with housework,
shopping, or babysitting. They can help with laundry, patient
transportation to outpatient clinics, and many other apparently
small but essential jobs.

The volunteer is also uniquely able to help the patient
maintain or reestablish a sense of self worth. Dependency and
lack of independent functioning created by disability eats away
at a person's self esteem. The withdrawal of health care professionals as they try to cope with their own feelings of inadequacy
reinforces the patient's diminishing sense of personhood. The
volunteer, by forming a close friendly relationship, can counter-
act this demeaning process.

We give volunteers a basic orientation to the program but do
not attempt to turn them into "counselors" for the dying. Their
special value is as a person with whom the patient can identify.
A patient sees them as "people like myself." Patients discuss
many areas with the lay volunteer that they do not discuss with
the professionals, either because they do not feel the doctor has
time to attend to these concerns, or because they believe the
doctor would not understand their position. For a low income
family, the volunteer who took the patient fishing was the only
person able to provide meaningful aid. Doctors, nurses, social
workers, psychiatric services had all been employed in attempts
to help the patient and family deal with their multiple problems.
All were consistently rejected. The only person who was accepted and helpful was the man who took him fishing and, in the
course of those trips, discussed at the same level on a person-to-
person basis the philosophies and fears the patient was encount-
ering. It is important to meet patients on their own ground.

Structured Personnel Support and
Communication Systems

Here is another area where much study needs to be done. From the 3 years of experience, we know that if personnel are to continue to form close human relationships (the foundations of hospice work), they must experience a kind of support not usually found in health care agencies. But within this general framework there are many unanswered questions. How should we select staff? Why do people come to work at Hospice? Why do they stay? Why do they leave? We have working opinions on these important matters and some functional approaches.

Quality inservice education, the team approach, administration-clinical communication, regular conferences (formal and informal), an occasional "day away" for all staff, a healthy volunteer corps, acceptance of grief and tears, monitoring work loads to prevent overzealous burnout syndrome, part-timers—these are just some of the mechanisms we use for staff support. Much needs to be learned.

Finances

Patients are accepted on the basis of health care need, not on ability to pay. No British hospice discriminates against patients because of their financial status, and American hospices must also strive to uphold this high standard of care. We cannot avoid our responsibility in this area by any references to socialized medicine. Most of the hospices in Britain are not under the National Health Service. Rather, they are financed by a combination of charitable donations, patient contributions, and government reimbursement.

Illustrative of the financial pain that can occur is the story of a patient who died this year, a 38-year-old man, a first generation Italian immigrant, husband and father of three children under 12 years of age. The patient had $12,000 in hospital bills that he was paying off at $50 a month. He owned his own home. He was too young for Medicare and too rich for Medicaid. He could have disposed of his assets to become eligible for Medicaid, but he and his wife were counting on their small family business and home to provide for the needs of their family after his death. This is just one example of the financial dilemma facing patients with a terminal illness.

There is a gaping void in our health care delivery system. Hospice has pioneered in developing a program that fills this void, ushering in a new kind of health care. This care has been accepted by the consumer and shown by objective study to improve the quality of life of patients with a terminal illness and their families.

References

1. Lack, S. A., Philosophy and organization of a hospice program. In Charles A. Garfield (Ed.), *Psychological care of the dying patient.* University of California School of Medicine, San Francisco, 1977.
2. Saunders, C. personal communication, May 1977.
3. Buckingham, R. W., & Lack, S. A. Final Report to National Cancer Institute, 1977.
4. Parkes, C. M., *Bereavement—studies of grief in adult life.* New York: International Universities Press, 1972.

Request reprints from Sylvia A. Lack, M.D., Hospice, Inc., 765 Prospect Street, New Haven, Conn. 06511.

MARIN COUNTY (1976)–DEVELOPMENT OF HOSPICE OF MARIN

WILLIAM M. LAMERS, JR.

University of California,
San Francisco

In 1974 a small group began an apparently inauspicious organization to provide more effective care of the terminally ill. Focus was to be on outpatient services, public and professional education, and institutional coordination.

Introduction

Marin County is a largely middle-class suburban community of slightly over 200,000 people, lying just north of San Francisco. Hospice of Marin is the result of repeated meetings during the early 1970s of three persons who became founding members of this hospice. They were a psychiatrist, a clergyman, and a homemaker. Each had numerous personal reasons to sense the need for change in existing social and medical support systems for dying patients and their families.

The founding members met in 1974 to explore the possibility of converting concern and talk into a new approach toward dying, death, and bereavement. The Hospice of Marin is a nonprofit organization that examined the needs of the dying. The standard of medical care was excellent; many organizations led by professionals and paraprofessionals provided a wide spectrum of services for the dying and their families. However, there was no coordination in some areas between those services that provided advice for funding and those services that provided helpers, both lay and professional, to do the work.

A survey of organizations that, in some way or another, dealt with dying patients and their families supported the impression that there was need for a hospice. Hospital administrators spoke of the inappropriateness of general hospitals for acute illnesses caring for the patients with terminal cancer, for whom a cure was no longer feasible.

Physicians spoke of the desire for an alternative to hospitalizing patients with terminal cancer. Families spoke of the frustration at being separated from their dying relative because they could not adequately care for them at home.

Early Organization

The initial board of three directors gradually grew to include several other interested professional and lay persons. In 1975 several charitable foundations were contacted to determine their interest in funding the planning phase of Hospice of Marin.

In the absence of early support from charitable foundations, expenses were kept to a minimum, and all hospice investigational and administrative activities were performed by lay and professional volunteers.

In late 1975 the decision was made to delay plans for development of an inpatient hospice facility and concentrate instead on delivering whatever services could be provided to a small number of patients, both to test the effectiveness of the hospice concept for care outside of an institution or facility, and to "develop a track record" that would provide experience for the hospice staff and evidence to the professional community of our intent to follow through on early planning.

Licensure, under the state laws of California, as a home health agency was obtained in early 1976. It was decided to hold publicity to a minimum in order to allow a gradual learning process to occur in lay and professional groups, and thereby avoid raising false or unrealistic expectations.

It was also decided at a very early point not to charge any fees for hospice care. Reasons for this included: (1) We hoped to be able to establish the practicality of hospice home care without having to focus on reimbursement; (2) we were concerned that if we developed a billing program along conventional lines, hospice care might not be seen as a unique addition to the medical care delivery system.

Education

At the beginning we learned that all of our previous professional education and experience was not sufficient to guarantee good hospice care for the dying. We had to learn new methods of controlling pain and symptoms in terminal illness. We had to come to better understandings of social, psychological, and spiritual aspects of death as they affected the dying person and the immediate family.

We had to learn to communicate more openly with each other and with the dying, their families, and the professional community.

At one point we estimated that about half of our early effort was spent in educating ourselves and then helping train the professional community. All those on the hospice staff participated in giving workshops, making speeches, and giving presentations describing the hospice and its activities to lay and professional groups in the surrounding areas. We taught courses at local colleges, taught postgraduate and continuing medical education courses for physicians and nurses, participated in seminars sponsored by the American Cancer Society, and addressed church groups and service organizations. We also attended training sessions and seminars on care of the terminally ill and assembled a library of printed and audio material to share both with each other and with new personnel on our staff.

Theory of Practice

We first wanted to avoid allowing dying to be a factor in fragmenting families. Drawing upon earlier hospice models, especially those in New Haven, Connecticut and London, we designed our program of care to make the patient and family the basic unit.

We tried to involve families in providing care, and now feel that the time we spent in providing instruction, supervision, and round-the-clock support to families resulted in patients receiving excellent care in comfortable surroundings.

We were, at times, amazed at the ability of families and friends to learn to give careful attention to skin care, bathing, oral hygiene, record-keeping, and general "comfort care." This participation showed us that the bereaved are able to show and give love, and to feel after the death that they were able to contribute something special during the last days of their loved one.

A second early concern was the lack of physician involvement with the dying patient. We saw evidence of the widespread phenomenon of physicians abandoning patients once cure was no longer possible. We hoped that by helping physicians learn more about practical aspects of terminal care, they would continue to have meaningful involvement with their patients and their families until the time of death.

Some physicians naturally continued to have good relationships with their patients and families until the time of death. Others gradually learned from our home care staff that there was always more that they could do to help provide comfort for the dying patient, or to help explain to the family what the course of illness might be.

During the early phase of our program, physician education took a considerable amount of time on the part of hospice staff physicians. It seemed essential to us that hospice care be carefully directed by a physician in order to develop a close, professional relationship with other physicians in the community involved. Although some physicians are open to suggestions from nurses and paraprofessionals, it is more expedient for physicians to communicate new skills to one another. This is especially true when dealing with a subject as complicated as pain control. Most physicians are skilled in the treatment of acute pain, but lacking in long-term management of chronic pain.

It is difficult to imagine providing hospice care without being intimately versed in the nuances of control of chronic pain. It is equally difficult to conceive of changing the way pain control is managed in any area served by a hospice unless a physician thoroughly knowledgeable in the hospice approach toward pain control is available to teach other physicians.

Third in our early considerations was our desire to convey in our hospice program the idea that death is a normal part of life. Herman Feifel (1) has told how, in our society, death that was once seen as a door to the hereafter has recently become a wall. We hoped that, by allowing families to become involved in the care of their dying loved one, they would be able to look at death in a more realistic way, and be less inclined to deny death, or suppress their feelings in reaction to death.

In part, families appeared to feel more comfortable with death by watching hospice personnel minister to their family member. Hospice personnel, through repeated contact with dying and death, tend to have a matter-of-fact attitude in talking about death, which makes it easier for dying patients to begin to talk about their own concerns.

It is also customary for hospice personnel to take an interest in funeral activities, and for those who are able, to attend funeral services.

Approach to Care

In most instances referrals to Hospice of Marin are made by the attending physician. The occasional direct referral from a family or friend must be followed by a request from the attending physician for the hospice to assist in care of the terminally ill patient.

One of the hospice staff nurses, usually the patient care coordinator, visits the patient as soon as possible to do an overall evaluation of suitability for hospice referral; to gather information from the patient/family and attending physician; and to begin formulating a treatment care plan, which is then reviewed with hospice medical staff.

Chronic pain is usually a predominant feature in patients referred for hospice care. It is impossible to do hospice work unless pain is controlled. Persistent or recurrent pain is usually accompanied by anxiety, depression, insomnia, and anorexia.

We now know that it is unnecessary for patients with

terminal cancer to endure chronic pain. The Brompton mixture, which was commonly used in England, has been replaced in the United States by a morphine-alcohol solution commonly known as "hospice mix." This combination of ingredients consists of morphine sulfate in a 20 percent alcohol solution, to which a flavoring agent and sugar solution is usually added.

If indicated, a phenothiazine such as Compazine or Thorazine may be added. Morphine, when given every 4 hours, is very effective in relieving chronic pain, even when administered orally, despite a long-standing prejudice against its medical usefulness.

When using narcotics on a regular basis, caution must be exercised to watch for side effects of constipation, nausea, and sedation. The side effect of sedation usually diminishes within the first 2 or 3 days of treatment. Side effects of nausea can be minimized by administering small amounts of Compazine. Constipation, if anticipated, can usually be treated with a combination of diet and stool softeners.

Proper medical management of symptoms that occur as a result of the terminal illness, or that arise from surgical, chemical, or radiation therapies directed at treatment of that illness, require individual assessment and treatment.

Once pain control is accomplished in coordination with the attending physician, and once the patient/family become comfortable with its increasing awareness of the possibility of controlling undesirable pain and physical symptoms, it is possible to begin looking at the patient's psychological, social, and spiritual concerns.

Family involvement and provision of this care make it less likely that communication and visiting barriers will arise. The patient/family is then actually one unit and attention of the attending physician and hospice staff can be directed toward that unit, rather than scattered among a number of people who do not communicate openly with each other.

It should be explained that, although we use the term *home care,* we also include patients who, for brief or even prolonged periods of time, reside in general hospitals or nursing homes in addition to their own homes.

The word *family* can also be interpreted rather loosely. One of the criteria for admission to the Hospice of Marin program is having a responsible care giver in the home. Several of our patients have lived alone in apartment units with no family member present to provide care. Yet they have been able to remain at home and be cared for by a surrogate family comprised of neighbors, friends, members of church groups, and members of service organizations, who come together to provide 24-hour coverage, support, and physical attention in the absence of family members.

Support for Care Givers

One of the Hospice of Marin staff nurses who served as a MASH nurse in Vietnam said, "Hospice work is more difficult than serving as a military surgical nurse in the field of combat." The difference, as Dr. Robert Fulton has pointed out (2), lies in the attachments that are formed between hospice personnel and the patient, as well as those formed between hospice nurses and the patients' families. These bonds are broken with the death of the patient, and hospice staff are left with their own grief. Unless the grief can be properly externalized, verbalized, communicated, and shared, enthusiasm for doing hospice work will soon lead to staff "burnout."

In the early days of the Hospice of Marin, each nurse in rotation was assigned to be "primary care nurse" for a new patient/family. After we became aware of the intensity of feelings involved in primary care nursing, we decided to change and have a team approach toward each patient/family. In this way, the intensity of feelings on the part of the team members was diminished and patients/families were less likely to feel disappointed if the primary nurse was otherwise occupied or on vacation.

We also learned from experience that it was unfair to expect nurses to work intensively in hospice home care for more than 4 full days per week. At 5 days per week, long hours of home visits, travel, record keeping, plus occasional night calls led to diminished motivation for hospice work. Once the level of work was reduced to 4 days per week, plus an occasional night or weekend call, the level of efficiency and attitude returned to an optimal level.

Hospice home care involves teamwork in another sense: The hospice team is multidisciplinary and should be cohesive, with excellent communication between all disciplines. The team at the Hospice of Marin consists of physicians, nurses, counselors (M.S.W. and marriage/family/child), an art therapist, a licensed home health aide, chaplains, a home care secretary, and a director of volunteers.

We have found it essential that the executive director of the overall hospice program attend weekly staff conferences in order to remain up to date with changing needs of program and personnel.

Bereavement

Those of us who have worked with dying patients one at a time have found it possible to maintain follow-up contact with families during bereavement. However, in a busy hospice program, it soon becomes difficult for staff to maintain contact with all bereaved families. This is one of the greatest conflicts we have faced in the development of Hospice of Marin. Occasional telephone calls and visits by hospice staff, plus remembrances at the time of the anniversary of the death, do not seem to be sufficient.

As a result, we have made several attempts to assist bereaved families. For example, identified "high risk" family members are referred to one of the hospice staff counselors for follow-up visits. At times, family members are referred to support persons and therapists in the community for individual or group counseling.

The Hospice of Marin also established a bereavement group, but found that this had only selective appeal for some of the survivors. Men especially were reluctant to attend the bereavement group where there were mainly women.

One of the problems inherent in this arrangement is the reluctance of family members to turn to staff who were not present during the time of terminal care at home. Staff nurses also expressed discontent at referring to third-party therapists family members with whom they had been close.

At present we are turning to families we have already served to ask for input in determining what, if anything, Hospice of Marin can do to assist during the bereavement period.

We are ready to explore the possibility of establishing a widow-to-widow program. What is definitely needed is further understanding of the bereavement process, based on observation, research, and analysis of bereavement models. Then it will be possible to develop a bereavement component of the hospice home care program that will be better able to meet the needs of survivors.

Conclusion

In an article in *Science,* Constance Holden (3) said, "The hospice program does not represent a new approach toward dying, but is simply an attempt to establish as standard those principles that have always guided the best practitioners." This statement should be amended because there are some things new about the hospice movement. Hospice is a medically directed, multidisciplinary team approach toward care of dying patients and their families. Hospice care implies a continuum ˙ from diagnosis, through terminal illness, to dying, and family bereavement.

Hospice care emphasizes total family involvement, and an openness of communications that is possible only if a cohesive staff providing 24-hour coverage can understand and meet the various needs of the patient/family. Hospice work requires special training and carries with it a responsibility to teach and train, in both professional and lay sectors.

If hospice care is to be more than a passing fad on the American medical scene, considerable work must be done to define carefully what hospice care is, determine who can best do hospice care, determine methods of reimbursement and, most of all, determine means of certifying hospice programs so that a standard of excellence, once begun, can be maintained.

62   *W. M. Lamers, Jr.*

References

1. Feifel, H. Death and dying in modern America. *Death Education*, 1977, *1*, 5–14.
2. Fulton, R. The sociology of death. *Death Education*, 1977, *1*, 15–25.
3. Holden, C. Hospices for the dying; relief from pain and fear. *Science*, 1976, *93*, 389–391.

Request reprints from Dr. William M. Lamers, Hospice of Marin, P.O. Box 72, Kentfield, Calif. 94904.

∞∞

TUCSON (1977)–HILLHAVEN HOSPICE

∞∞

JOHN A. HACKLEY
The Hillhaven Foundation, Tacoma, Washington

WILLIAM C. FARR and Sr. TERESA MARIE McINTIER
Hillhaven Hospice, Tucson, Arizona

Hillhaven Hospice began patient services in 1977 as the nation's first "free standing," comprehensive service hospice. This paper is a description of how the program was designed to be part of a community's total health system, how it is staffed, and what its principles are.

Introduction

Hillhaven Hospice in Tucson, Arizona is, in 1977, the nation's only autonomous hospice to offer a comprehensive program of care. Its range of services for terminal cancer patients includes care in the home, day care at the hospice, 24-hour inpatient care in 19 semiprivate rooms and 1 private room, and a 12-month bereavement service for the family following death of a patient. The hospice, which began offering care April 17, 1977, was developed by and is totally an operation of The Hillhaven Foundation in Tacoma, Washington.

Assessment of the need for, and feasibility of, a hospice, as well as subsequent program planning, began in 1975 and continued for 2 years. Throughout this long period of planning and preparation, The Hillhaven Foundation collaborated with several community and state health planning, service, and reimbursement agencies as well as with the University of Arizona's College of Medicine, Arizona Health Sciences Center, College of Nursing,

College of Pharmacy, and College of Business and Public Administration. Prior to construction, the hospice was granted a certificate of need for long-term care beds and is currently licensed by the state as a certified nursing care facility. However, The Hillhaven Foundation is applying for licensing and recognition as a "special hospital-hospice." A special bed category has been established in the state plan by the Health Systems Agency of Southeastern Arizona and special licensure regulations are being developed by the state health department.

The Hillhaven Hospice is designed to serve dying patients with an array of services modeled as closely as possible after the pioneering St. Christopher's Hospice in London, which was developed by Dr. Cicely Saunders.

The Hillhaven Hospice provides a program of service to dying patients for whom active therapeutic treatment is no longer being aggressively pursued or deemed appropriate. Its medically directed program offers palliative and supportive care to terminally ill patients and their families in collaboration with the patients' attending physician. Essentially, the goal of the hospice is to provide patients and their families with as tranquil, supportive, and dignified an experience as possible.

This program is intended to create hospice care as part of existing community health care systems. The Hillhaven Hospice creates a program model with features of outreach to referring hospital or physician, home care, adult day health care, inpatient services, and after-care for families of the deceased patient.

Future research efforts of Hillhaven Hospice will address the effects of a hospice on a community health care system. An evaluative research component will provide documentation for service development, utilization, and effectiveness of such services on a nationwide basis.

At present, implementation of the hospice program in the context of an existing community service network affords responses to key issues on the role of the medical profession, integration of hospice into existing health care networks, and outcome in terms of family and individual patient care. The major function of the program is the enhancement of the quality of life, particularly for terminally ill patients and their families.

During the past few years, the thrust of institutional health care has been on rehabilitation, restoration, and current approaches to development of human potential. However, based both on national and Hillhaven Foundation statistics of discharge rates and reasons, this focus appears to be inappropriate for the needs of 30 percent of all nursing home patients who die in a year.

Emphasis on restoration has had an impact on staff who provide care for the terminally ill. In an environment where rehabilitation receives major attention, death may communicate personal and professional failure to staff, thus affecting morale, performance, and turnover rate. This rehabilitation emphasis also communicates failure to families and residents of older persons, often creating a sense that dying is "inappropriate." There has been a tendency nationally for quality of nursing home care to be based on discharge rates due to death. Consequently, nursing homes and physicians have been subtly encouraged to transfer patients, often during the final days of life, into institutional acute care settings.

The Hillhaven Foundation, in its educational programs, has become increasingly aware of the need for programs of service planned particularly for the terminally ill. The foundation staff has found that the hospice care model is the only potentially multifaceted program for offering both assistance to the terminally ill and support for staff to contribute personally and professionally to the needs of dying persons and their families in an enlightened and satisfying way.

Purpose

The Hillhaven Hospice program is designed to fill gaps in existing service to the terminally ill patient without unnecessary duplication. Because of the very personal impact of cancer on the patient and family, the program must be sensitive and flexible to specific needs. To this end some of the objectives of the program are to:

1. Maintain the terminally ill patient in the home until death, or as long as possible, by providing home health

services, outpatient day or night care, and all of the expertise of the hospice staff for consultation and treatment.

2. Provide day or night care services for those patients who might otherwise have to be admitted to the inpatient facility for lack of suitable care arrangements at home.
3. Provide consultation services to the community for symptom control problems.
4. Provide an inpatient facility that is designed and operated to meet the total needs of dying patients and their families.
5. Provide educational experiences on terminal care for community professionals.
6. Study the impact of the hospice program on care of the terminally ill patient and the family in the Tucson community.
7. Consider not only the patient but the family and significant others as part of the unit to which supportive services are offered.
8. Ensure that major emphasis is placed on the care giver being sensitive to the patient's needs, comforts, and desires.
9. Maintain and respect the important role played by the primary attending physician with the service of the hospice being supportive to the physician.
10. Help coordinate and facilitate the use of available community services in the program, for example, the American Cancer Society, local transportation, Meals on Wheels.
11. Provide bereavement services to the family for at least 1 year after the death of the patient.
12. Be willing to learn from our patients and families.
13. Provide the service in a free standing facility under the auspices of a nonprofit foundation.

Program and Services

The hospice is not a facility of brick and mortar but a continuum of care for the terminally ill cancer patient. Its four phases are (1) home health care, (2) outpatient day or night care, (3) inpatient care, and (4) a bereavement program for the surviving family.

A suitable patient to be enrolled in the hospice program is someone with terminal cancer within six months of death. Ideally the patient is referred to the program early enough to benefit from the many services available—before the last few days of life. A referral may be useful to the physician or family for the coordination of services to the terminally ill. An appropriate referral is for evaluation and consultation for pain and symptom control. Bereavement counseling for the family after the patient's death is available from the hospice.

Once admitted to the hospice program, the patient may move into the various levels of care without the need for application and a lot of paperwork. Only patients with private physicians are admitted to the program and it is our philosophy that the private attending physician remains the cornerstone of care of the patient through all phases of the illness.

Home Health Services

Home health services at present are provided by the Visiting Nurse Association of Tucson. The hospice staff coordinates this care with the Visiting Nurse Association and supplements care when necessary, particularly at night and on weekends when the association does not serve. An attempt is made to maintain the patient at home through the terminal phase of illness. Only after home care is less than adequate for the patient and/or family will a recommendation be made for transfer to day care or the inpatient facility.

Outpatient Day or Night Care

Outpatient day or night care can serve a useful function to the family and patient when vital family members can no longer be in attendance 24 hours a day. The patients may be brought to the hospice for several hours a day. They will receive food, medication, lodging, and nursing care, plus all other services available to the inpatient. In this way, family members may be "freed" of their patient care responsibilities and have time for social or business outings or just time off.

Inpatient Care

Once it has been ascertained that the patient can no longer be managed in the home environment, he or she is admitted to the hospice inpatient facility. This facility has 39 beds. At present, it is licensed as a certified nursing facility with more services than required of such a facility. The staff is trained in the care of the dying and are qualified to evaluate the symptom control programs of the physicians.

Supportive Services

Available in all levels of the program is physical therapy, social services, occupational therapy, dietary services, a chaplain, and counseling services. There is a clinical pharmacist who reviews drug regimes on a regular basis and is of assistance to the physician, the patient, and the family in the areas of pharmaceutical education both in the facility and at home.

Counseling Services

Hillhaven Hospice provides its patients and their families with several different types of counseling services. Such supportive therapy may take the form of the nursing staff simply talking or listening. More formal supportive care is provided on an ongoing basis by the facilitator and the medical social worker. The latter conducts weekly group meetings for the families and patients. In conjunction with the above program, the director of creative communications has been using art and poetry as a medium through which the patient and family may express their feelings in a therapeutic way. As death approaches an attempt is made to foster meaningful and healthy dialogue when necessary.

Formal psychiatric counseling is available through private community resources. Tucson East Community Mental Health Center and Dr. Stephen Shanfield of the University of Arizona

Psychiatry Department provide consulting psychiatric services to the hospice staff and to some patients.

Bereavement Services

The families of patients who die while enrolled in a hospice program have available to them counseling and follow-up support for a period of at least 1 year after the patient's death. The hospice periodically calls upon the willing family after the death until it is clear that no additional service is needed.

Physician Services

Physician services within the Hillhaven Hospice are provided for by each patient's attending physician in conjunction with the hospice medical director. Participation of the medical director is not intended to exclude or compromise the importance of the patient's existing relationship with the attending physician. The supervision and specialized experience of the hospice physician is provided as a service to ensure continuous monitoring of the treatment plan and as an effort to provide the most comprehensive, compassionate care plan possible. The medical director, in this capacity, is able to keep the attending physician abreast of the latest developments in the patient's condition and treatment.

Referral to the Hospice Program

Referral to the hospice program can be made by almost anyone. Referrals are taken from physicians, social workers, agencies, families, and patients. In all circumstances, no matter who makes the referral, the consent of the attending physician is necessary for admission into the program.

All that is required is that one phone the hospice and express interest in referring a patient. The referral is given to the facilitator, who contacts the primary physician to obtain the necessary medical information and approval of the patient's entrance into the program. The facilitator then visits the family and the patient and obtains the medical record. Once the patient is admitted, the facilitator, the medical director, and the primary physician, along with the family and the patient, will decide on the appropriate level of care and the necessary strategy to implement the service.

The Hospice Staff

The Medical Director

The specific duties of the medical director include but are not necessarily restricted to the following:

1. Supervising and operating the hospice as well as directing the care programs.
2. Providing direct patient care in conjunction with the attending physician.
3. Visiting each patient and reviewing the care plan with the staff.
4. Ensuring that the appropriate modalities of treatment are offered for pain and symptom relief.
5. Making recommendations and writing orders on the dosage of analgesics, antiemetics, psychotropic drugs, and others when needed (no new medications or stop orders are made without first consulting the attending physician).
6. Making recommendations to the attending physician on modalities of treatment that are seemingly appropriate and conveying suggestions for changes in the treatment plan offered by the patient care committee.
7. Providing an ongoing education for the community at large and making available to physicians within the community those accomplishments deemed worthwhile in the care of the terminally ill.
8. Acting as spokesperson for the hospice in the community.
9. Coordinating the educational programs for the staff.

The Nurse

Nursing care is directed toward assisting each patient to achieve the level of self-care and independence that is needed to live fully and die with dignity. Although the physical care of the patient receives scrupulous attention, the psychoemotional dimension consumes more time. In the resolution of unfinished business, the terminal patient requires both time to sort out feelings and a person who is willing to listen and willing to share. The nurse communicates with the patient in a variety of ways, by providing information, explanation, or instruction. The nurse will also use conversation as a therapeutic tool to allay apprehension and thereby enhance the patient's comfort. Communication is also employed as a vehicle for diversion.

Whatever the method, nurses do more than merely exchange words. They interchange understood meanings. This implies in-depth conversation. They not only use knowledge about cancer as an illness but also come to grips with their own feelings about pain, loss, death, and helplessness. When a patient is too ill or depressed to talk, nurses may speak volumes by tender care, explaining each procedure, or may be found sitting quietly by the bed. To meet the many and varied needs of the terminally ill, nurses move closer to their patients and risk a certain amount of discomfort. When they assuage the pain of loneliness, they realize they no longer work alone but, together, nurses and patients surmount obstacles neither could alone.

The Chaplain

The patients—Christians, Jews, Buddhists, Native Americans with special beliefs, and those with no religious affiliation come to the hospice. Patients entering the hospice are received as a child of God no matter what their religious beliefs are. The hospice respects the right of each person to worship or not, according to personal choice.

When patients are admitted to the hospice, an effort is made to determine their religious affiliations. A patient's local minister is advised of admission if the patient wishes. The minister may then maintain a close relationship with a patient during the hospice stay. When the patient nears death the minister is notified immediately.

The hospice chaplain maintains a supportive relationship with all patients. Spiritual and/or emotional problems are identified and dealt with. It is not unusual for a patient to deny the existence of cancer upon admission to the hospice. Nor is it unusual for the patient to maintain this defense by saying, for example, "I had cancer but my 25 radiation treatments cleared it. I will be here only until I get stronger and then I will go home." This defense is needed until the patient is ready to move on to the next step toward acceptance of the illness.

There is anger among the patients as well as among the family. A husband and wife may plan a suicidal pact involving both before death by cancer makes its claim. A spouse may promise to commit suicide as soon as the other dies (or may agree to try it alone for a year to see how it goes before committing suicide). Emotions play a major role in the lives of dying cancer patients and their families. The hospice staff is aware of the emotional impact of cancer on them and support these troubled people with love, compassion, and understanding.

Patients and families who move toward an acceptance of the reality of cancer and impending death may demonstrate this acceptance by jointly preparing the funeral service or by making certain requests of the chaplain concerning the upcoming funeral. This preparation helps patient and family accept the inevitable.

Many patients have unfinished business to take care of such as seeing a certain relative or friend, making amends for a wrong doing, or even taking a joy ride in a helicopter. The hospice staff encourages the patient to take care of unfinished business and they help facilitate this when necessary so that the patient may die comfortably and in peace.

Within the hospice is a nondenominational chapel for use by patients, families, and friends for meditation and prayer. It may also be used by the clergy for worship with their patients, families, and hospice community. Adjacent to the chapel is a viewing room where the deceased may lie on a bed surrounded by family members who may desire a few moments of privacy with their loved one. They may wish to touch the deceased again and say affectionate goodbyes.

The chaplain provides the opportunity for individual religious expression related to the needs of the terminally ill and the family unit. This involves reporting to the hospice team on the specific religious practices of the individual, providing input to the patient's minister and planning with the patient and family minister a meaningful spiritual response to the needs of the patient. The hospice chaplain is neither a provider nor a promoter of any single religion or religious practice, but rather a representative of, and link to, the religious community for the patient and the staff. The hospice chaplain also assists in the education program to assure that staff and volunteers have an understanding of religious practices related to the patients they are serving.

The Facilitator

Hospice care of the patient and family begins with a visit from the facilitator, who is a registered nurse with a master's degree in counseling and guidance. The facilitator assesses all patients prior to admission and arranges for appropriate services within the hospice program with consultation from other team members. The facilitator has one of the key roles in the entire hospice program and is the advocate for the patient and family throughout the length of time the service is provided them.

Following the death of a patient, the facilitator activates the system of continued assistance to provide comfort, guidance, and information as desired by the family throughout the process of grieving and bereavement. This family program continues for the period of 1 year following the patient's death and consists of assistance toward emotional, personal, social, physical, and economic adjustment to death.

The Pharmacist

The hospice clinical pharmacist develops, coordinates, and supervises all pharmaceutical services, which include those of the home care, day and night care, and inpatient segments of hospice.

Initially it was essential to develop policies and procedures for the pharmaceutical services that complied with state and federal regulations and fit into the hospice concept. As Hillhaven Hospice continues to grow, it will be necessary to continually re-evaluate the policies and procedures and to adapt them to the changes.

The clinical pharmacist is available to those patients at home and their families to educate them on the patient's medication. A thorough discussion of the drug treatment plan is made, including personal reinforcement and instructions on how to take and store medications. The visiting nurses and others who work with the patients in their homes also call upon the pharmacist at any time with drug-related questions.

The education and discussion regarding drug treatment plans are also available to patients and family members while in the hospice facility. During these discussions the clinical pharmacist, both subjectively and objectively, evaluates the effects or side effects of medications being used and coordinates this information with other members of the staff to ensure quality care for the patient.

At the time of admission, the clinical pharmacist performs an intake review of the patient's drug regimen and follows with continual monitoring of it, which allows the clinical pharmacist to assist in choosing optimum drug regimens and making necessary dosage adjustments when indicated to optimize effect while decreasing side effects. These decisions are made by direct contact with the physician, with the nursing staff or in the weekly patient care meetings.

The clinical pharmacist also monitors record keeping in order to assure the control of all drugs. Any irregularities are reported to the nursing staff, administration, or medical director.

Education of all members of the hospice staff is an important role of the clinical pharmacist. It includes both educating the nursing staff on policies and procedures for all aspects of pharmaceutical services, inservice programs, and being available as a source of drug information on a one-to-one basis.

Interwoven within all activities is the opportunity for pharmacy students to learn about hospice and the hospice concept, dying patients, cancer and its treatment, pain and its treatment, and, of great importance, how to communicate with the terminally ill.

Volunteers

Hillhaven Hospice, like other health care centers, graciously accepts the supportive services of a group of volunteers. Hospice volunteers come from virtually every level on the socioeconomic scale. They are actively engaged in volunteer work and receive no financial assistance. Volunteers range in age from 16 to over 80. Their services extend from 2 through 14 hours per week. Tasks are performed at specific times from 2 to 4 hours on a regular basis.

The educational backgrounds of volunteers vary. Our statistics suggest that willingness to volunteer is directly proportional to a higher degree of education. Professionals tend to express their wishes to work in the capacity of their educational backgrounds. The hospice grants this opportunity.

The primary areas for volunteer involvement are (1) administrative assistants, (2) activity assistants, and (3) assistants in patient care. Since the participants of every group work in accordance with their skills and personal preference, each person's contribution of time and effort is valued equally. Thus, the following positions in the area of administrative assistance are crucial at Hillhaven Hospice. Adequate coverage through volunteer work enables hospice personnel to render high quality professional care to patients. Volunteers may work as receptionists, operators, supply coordinators, messengers, or typists, and may be involved in a wide variety of duties, e.g., xeroxing, addressing, labeling, or filing.

In the area of activities, anyone with special talents can shine! Hospice patients still value old-fashioned home cooking, hence we have bakers, cooks, and candymakers among our volunteers who prepare small, appetizing portions for our patients whose appetites are often lacking. There are volunteers who assist in transporting the patients to a weekly "happy hour," who play minimum exertion games, who sing, perform, or play instruments, who read and entertain. Some volunteers assist in the various activities at the hospice. There are some volunteers who are eager to learn from the occupational therapist and help patients with short-term arts and crafts projects, while others gather materials and act as decorators for holidays and birthday parties.

Volunteer services in the area of patient care were initially viewed with great skepticism. Would the volunteer professionals render quality care and could untrained people be expected to help with nursing tasks? We found that there was no general answer and that we could only rely upon intuition and personal judgment. Those volunteers who have worked with our patients consider it a privilege. Everyone is quickly "infected" with hospice goals and philosophies and value the harmonious environment. Volunteers make friendly visits, act as go-betweens with libraries and audio-video services, help patients with their correspondence, and assist the nursing staff with simple care tasks.

One cannot overlook those volunteers with special talents who work independently outside of the above three groups. There is, for example, the person who transports and repairs televisions free of charge as long as parts are available; the cosmetologist who realizes the importance of self-image and spends many hours of free time dressing our patients' hair; and the flutists, guitarists, and gentle singers who drop by once a week, simply to add some cheer to our peaceful world.

Hospice volunteers are drawn from the community. Their desire to serve is often based on a recent loss among their friends or relatives. They wish that the hospice had been there when they needed it. However, there are other reasons for volunteering at the hospice that are coupled with society's changing view about death and deep-seated religious beliefs that make each and every one of us kin to the dying patient.

Family

An important goal of the hospice is to strengthen and maintain family ties. This goal is best achieved through a family-centered approach to care. Such an avenue provides special consideration for children. In the acute health care setting, children are often restricted from visiting hospitalized family members. Fortunately this is not the case in the hospice. It is a unique experience to be emotionally and intellectually aware of the death process and at the same time to hear the joyful laughter and delighted voices of children ring through the corridors.

Fond (1) believes that, "in families, no matter how extended or nuclear, every member plays an important and unique role." Children bring love and sunshine not only into the life of a family member but to all the patients in the hospice.

Since one's attitudes about death are learned, the staff believes that the children who are permitted to visit the terminal patient and observe the interaction between staff and patient will form healthy attitudes about death and loss.

A 4-year-old frequently visited her grandmother in the hospice. She would sing and dance to "make Grandma happy." One day Becky skipped down to the nurse's station and said she knew a secret. She then announced, "My Grandma's going to heaven and she's starting out here."

On another occasion an 8-year-old was attentively observing the nurses transport a recently deceased patient to the viewing room. When the nurse emerged from the room with an empty bed, the child asked if he could help wheel it back. En route he commented to the nurse, "You just sent someone to heaven, didn't you?" Regan (2) believes, "Within a professional role, the nurse can be a trusted confidant on whom the family and child rely for emotional support, not heroic measures once all hope is gone" (pp. 666–667).

The hospice staff directs the crisis of death toward a quiet resolution for all family members—seeing each member as a unique individual.

In designing the care plan, the nurse allows for family relationships and responsibilities, keeping them within the framework of the coping capabilities of the family. Fond (1) submits that, "in time, the activities and family position of the absent individual may be taken over by another member, but at the time of loss, the balance is disturbed sufficiently to necessitate health appraisal and, perhaps, intervention" p. 54.

Providing skilled care without sacrificing the companionship of family members sets the hospice apart from the usual health care facilities. Institutional routines are set aside in favor of the patient's involvement and control of the surrounding environment. Family members are important and are encouraged to contribute information about the patient's dietary preferences and sleep and activity patterns. With this information a plan of care is designed to meet the individual needs of each patient.

The "Little" Extras

Flexibility

The hospice has to meet the needs of the patient and family in a way that is meaningful and in a home-like atmosphere. To this end, visiting hours are any time and family members of all ages, including favorite pets, are allowed to visit. When necessary, the family is encouraged to stay with the patient at all times and sleeping accommodations and meals within the facility are arranged.

Dietary Services

We feel a need for maximum flexibility in dietary services. Three large meals a day are often not desired by the terminal patient. We provide a selective menu. The food not eaten, but desired at a later time, can be stored on the ward and reheated. A special kitchen in the facility is available to the patient and family at all times for dining together or for the family to make or reheat a home-cooked meal. No dietary request is too small and an attempt is made to obtain whatever the patient wants. A consultant dietitian is available to all patients.

The Moving Bed

The patients are encouraged to socialize and to move about the facility, taking advantage of our occupational therapy and creative writing instructor, crafts, or just enjoying the out-of-doors. Patients unable to ambulate or be transported in a wheelchair can have their beds moved easily inside or outside the facility. We even have a golf cart that picks patients up at their doors in order to take them for rides around the grounds.

Creative Communications

Communication is important, whether it be between the patient and loved ones or with the staff, a friend, or a significant person of religious faith. Our social worker, facilitator, chaplain, and creative communications director attempt to foster significant communication when it seems necessary. We boldly thought about methods to improve communication early in our experience with the dying patient. Counseling in a traditional sense seems inappropriate at times for the dying patient. Thus we have turned to the arts in attempts to approach communication. Our communications director has a background in psychology, poetry, and art. He is guiding our patients and their families with interesting results. Through sharing his knowledge of the arts, we have found expressions with feelings and have observed some very meaningful and reflective messages.

A Word about Terminality

Admission to the program does not require that the patient be fully informed of his diagnosis or prognosis. Most of us would agree that a patient should be told but occasionally there are sound reasons to delay the discussion of prognosis. This should be communicated at the time of referral.

At the hospice, terminality is neither dwelled upon nor ignored. We cannot lie, our patients let us know in different ways when, what, and how much is to be said. Our objective is a healthy approach to coming to terms with dying. This very special and individual experience may take days or weeks, but in each case the individual, through words and actions, is able to set the timetable.

Pain Control Program

Patients admitted to the hospice program are maintained on the care plan offered by their attending physicians. During the first

24 to 48 hours after admission, the effectiveness of the program for pain control is evaluated by the nursing staff and the medical director. Lack of success is reported to the attending physician with suggestions offered by the medical director. An attempt is made to provide pain relief by the use of a preventive dosage schedule (as suggested by Dr. Cicely Saunders).

We try to provide analgesics orally until no longer viable because of difficulty in swallowing. Our analgesic preference to date is the modified Brompton mixture, which contains morphine sulfate, water, and grenadine syrup. We have found this to be effective, generally nonsedating, palatable, and relatively inexpensive. Our success parallels that reported by Cicely Saunders and Robert Twycross at St. Christopher's Hospice in London.

In addition, patients receive palliative chemotherapy or radiation therapy as a part of their pain control program when so dictated by the course of the disease. This is generally the exception rather than the rule for patients who are involved in the inpatient facility since they are usually more ill and, consequently, closer to death.

Newsletter

Hillhaven Hospice has two newsletters. One was developed by the staff with contributions from patients and families. This newsletter is circulated periodically within the program and goes to patients and their families.

Our second is a medical newsletter prepared by the medical director and staff on terminal care. This is circulated to community physicians and health related agencies. The medical newsletter also serves as a forum where questions can be posed by those serving terminal patients in the community. The answers are sought from community and hospice resources. Also, articles are solicited on terminal care techniques from community resources for inclusion in the newsletter.

Conclusion

Thus far, exploration about feasibility of hospice services in the United States has taken three approaches to the replication of

St. Christopher's: (1) free standing, (2) hospital based, and (3) home care oriented. Inasmuch as over 90 percent of the current hospice program efforts in the United States are still, in late 1977, in the planning and early developmental phases, it is obvious that there will not be adequate operational and outcome data to attest to which approach is preferable if, indeed, any one single approach can ever be deemed so. Hillhaven has followed the "free standing" approach.

Inasmuch as Hillhaven Hospice included the 24-hour-a-day inpatient care component from its inception, the inpatient portion of the hospice program began as a certified-skilled nursing care facility. In the judgment of the official regulatory agency, this was the obvious "nonacute" licensure category in existence that most closely approximated the hospice program. Subsequently, with the assistance of the Health Systems Agency of Southeastern Arizona, in collaboration with the Arizona State Departments of Health Services and Social Welfare, a special category was established within the State Hillburton Plan titled, "Special Hospital-Hospice" in order that a unique licensure code and special regulations could be developed that could apply to the unique nature of this program.

Whatever a community's or region's approach to assessment of need and development of a comprehensive hospice program, it is essential that the planning and development body fully realize that there will inevitably be compromises between the prototype hospice program of St. Christopher's Hospice and what is feasible in any one community or locality in the United States. Once that is accepted, it is incumbent upon the planning group to accept only unavoidable compromises that least jeopardize the basic components of hospice philosophy and concepts.

In a program such as that of Hillhaven Hospice, which is generally referred to as "free standing," there is a greater component of community orientation than in either of the other two current modes. This community orientation of a hospice program provides a comprehensive community organization feature for both assessment of community needs and determination of hospice feasibility within the prescribed area. It also opens up extra-ordinarily beneficial avenues for community involvement, liaisons with existing health and social care resources, and provides for continued comprehensive community involvement in the ongoing conduct of the hospice program.

In order that a hospice program conceived for a particular community or region be fiscally sound to endure, there must be adequate measurable need for the full array of hospice services, adequate health personnel of the unique kinds and qualities a hospice program requires, and substantial comprehensive clinical resources for oncological services for diagnosis, assessment, and treatment available within the same service area. Hospice care is not a substitute for aggressive therapeutic and curative efforts but rather provides a program of palliative care after all of the reasonable potentials of aggressive treatment have been exhausted.

One major opposition to hospices held by some leading oncologists in the United States is based upon fear that some programs will be so preoccupied with efforts to help patients die they will inadvertently thwart the patient and family from living as well as they could during the patient's last period of life. If one admits that these United States have long been characterized by the fadist approach to health care, then one can also recognize that there may be, on occasion, some justification for such apprehension.

It has been said that one interpretation of health is the degree of wellness possessed by the person and that this degree of wellness is understood to be the best compromise that can be achieved between the patient and the illness. No doubt, in the context of hospice, this definition would relate to the best degree of compromise that can be achieved between the patient/family and the terminal nature of the illness.

References

1. Fond, K. I. Dealing with death and dying through family-centered case. *Nursing Clinics of North America,* 1977, 7(1).
2. Regan, P. The dying person and his family. *Journal of the American Medical Association,* 1965, *192,* 666–667.
3. McCaffery, M. *Nursing management of the patient with pain.* Philadelphia: Lippincott, 1972.

Request reprints from John A. Hackley, president, The Hillhaven Foundation, P.O. Box 11222, Tacoma, Wash. 98411.

∞∞

SPRINGFIELD (1978)–ST. JOHN'S HOSPICE

∞∞

JAMES COX

Southern Illinois University, Springfield

Springfield, Illinois is planning a hospice to care for the terminally ill. It is not intended to be restricted to either geriatric or cancer patients. St. John's Hospital, together with the Southern Illinois University School of Medicine's Departments of Family Practice and Medical Humanities, have joined together to develop plans.

Emphasis will be on quality of life for the patient, with attention focused on physical, social, psychological, and spiritual needs. Care will be provided both in the hospice and at home, with emphasis on helping patients and families to help each other. The unit will also be used for the education of medical students, residents, and other health professionals.

The inpatient unit will have 20–25 beds, with two beds per room. Patients will be encouraged to bring their personal belongings with them and there will be a liberal visiting policy. To build continuity and trust, a team of physician, nurse, and patient and family support personnel will be provided for each patient. An unlisted telephone hot line for the support of patients and families at home will be operated continuously.

Some of the problems encountered so far are described.

Introduction

Like many communities throughout the United States, Springfield, Illinois is in the process of developing a hospice. Springfield has a population of 100,000 and is the state capital. It has three hospitals, two of which are affiliated with Southern Illinois University School of Medicine. The school of medicine is committed to improvement of primary care for the people of central and southern Illinois.

83

St. John's Hospital, founded in 1875 by the Hospital Sisters of the Third Order of St. Francis, is one of the largest Catholic operated hospitals in the United States. The hospital has 670 acute care beds as well as a recently purchased 232 bed long-term care facility in which the hospice will be housed.

In our planning we benefitted considerably from the experience of other pioneers in this field, both through the literature and by direct communication and encouragement. A description of our approach to the problem of caring for dying patients and their families might be of help to those in other places struggling with the same problems.

The Need

Over the last decade countless words have been written about death and dying, highlighting the increasing awareness of the deficiencies in our care of the terminally ill (1-4). There is no doubt that there is a need for improved care of the dying, but unfortunately the United States seems to be lagging behind Great Britain and Canada in this field (5-7). In Springfield, the need for change is neither greater nor less than the need for change anywhere else in the United States. In fact, Springfield may have a head start over some similar communities for three reasons. First, St. John's Hospital Pastoral Care Department has for a long time provided emotional and spiritual support to dying patients and their families. Help at the time of crisis is followed up by care of the bereaved for as long as they need it, which includes a monthly service for bereaved families and a message of remembrance on the anniversary of a patient's death. Second, the department of medical humanities in the school of medicine has since its inception provided support and assistance in the care of dying patients in both of Springfield's major hospitals. Third, some of Springfield's physicians have for many years felt the need for improved palliative care of their dying patients.

The need for educating medical students and other health professionals in the care of the terminally ill has frequently been identified by the students and their teachers and counselors. One of our medical students, describing an experience with a dying patient, wrote

> To most of my patients, going home was the end of their problems, but for Mr. K., going home would be the beginning of a downhill course. It seemed that we had little in common, little to talk about, so my daily visits were brief. Never once did I initiate a discussion concerning his feelings about the situation. He seemed less depressed, seemed to be adjusting, and I felt inadequately prepared to offer him anything more. And so, I cared for his physical needs until he was discharged from my care.

Historical Background

Four years ago three senior nurses from St. John's decided that they would like to hold some workshops on death and dying. They sought the help of the sister in charge of pastoral care, whose daily work brought her into contact with the dying and their relatives and who was well aware of the hospice concept. Considerable enthusiasm was generated throughout the order and there was some suggestion that an oncology unit be established within the hospital. Unfortunately, many of the staff, including physicians, saw such a unit as a depressing, deadly place where everyone would be unhappy, gloomy, and dying. That such a unit would cross traditional specialty borders was also seen as a problem. However, in due course an "oncology task force" proposed that an "oncology nurse" be appointed and that this person's duties should include visiting patients and consulting with other nurses regarding cancer patients' problems.

This nurse was appointed in August 1976. She had experience in the care of patients with malignant disease and was aware of their need to talk. She had already discovered while on night duty that if one talks and listens to patients they require fewer analgesic drugs or sedatives. Given flexible guidelines to her responsibilities, she has filled a need by visiting cancer patients throughout the hospital. She works closely with patients' families and with nurses in direct contact with the patients, and is able to help patients and their families come to terms with their illnesses. She receives referrals from staff (although from few physicians) and from the list of hospital admissions.

In 1975–1976, St. John's Hospital undertook an extensive long-range planning process involving 220 physicians and 100 hospital employees and community leaders. During the process, the planners were addressed by an appeal from the hospital's pastoral care department to consider the specialized needs of terminally ill patients. This appeal was endorsed by the school of medicine's department of medical humanities, which was already involved in care of terminally ill patients. The decision regarding acquisition of a 232 bed long-term care facility by the hospital, which made new beds available for the development of a hospice, was further encouraged by the school of medicine's department of family practice, which sees management of terminally ill patients and their families as part of family care.

Planning for the potential creation of a hospice within the long-term care facility was begun in earnest in March 1977. In June 1977 the planning and development committee of the hospital decided to go ahead with development of such a unit. The Hospice Planning Committee is advisory to the administration of the hospital. To make it workable, we have attempted to keep it small. Its membership consists of representatives from the pastoral care, nursing, and planning departments of the hospital, and representatives from the departments of family practice and medical humanities of the medical school.

Current Plans

The long-term care facility purchased by the hospital was formerly a 4-story nursing home with 232 beds. The whole facility is licensed by the state for skilled nursing care, and the hospital's intention is that approximately half of the beds should be used for postacute skilled nursing care. None of the beds is licensed as acute medical or surgical bed. The remainder of the facility will include a physical rehabilitation unit, an adult day-care unit, a home health care program, and the hospice. The hospice will have 20–25 beds, occupying half of one floor. There is a large conference/dining room on each floor, which will be used for communal patient and family activity. Because we feel that it is preferable that the views from the windows of the hospice rooms give a feeling of life and activity, we have recommended that the unit overlook the busy hospital, rather than a more peaceful wooded area, even if this carries with it the risk of more disturbance from noise.

There has been considerable discussion here, as in most hospices that exist or are being planned, about the optimum number of beds that should be in each room. This facility has two beds per room and since this could not be altered without considerable expense, our discussion has been purely academic! However, some of the points to consider are interesting. Single-bed rooms tend to isolate patients and are generally undesirable. There are exceptions. For example, a private room may be preferable for a business person who wishes to work while in the hospice, or it may be necessary for a patient whose physical condition is intolerable for other patients. A two-bed room places a heavy burden upon the patient who survives, and a three-bed room often results in two of the patients building up a close relationship and one being left out. But in a three-bed room, when one patient dies the survivors can support each other. It may be that to have four-bed rooms would present the least problems (8). Unfortunately, it is not possible here.

We plan to provide home care using, if possible, the same personnel that will be involved in inpatient and day care, taking advantage of the physical therapy and other facilities available in the building. To have the same nurses providing both inpatient and home care may not be feasible but we will attempt it in order to provide continuity of care for patients. However, some nurses work best independently and may be suited to home care while others work better as part of a team. It may not be possible for a nurse (or anyone else) to do both well, and we may have to abandon the idea.

The intention is that, wherever possible, patients should be cared for at home by their own family with the support of the staff from the hospice. The day care and inpatient services will therefore be aimed at educating patients and their families, as well as providing an environment for skilled nursing care and relief of pain. The objectives of the hospice are listed as follows:

1. *Care of the Terminally Ill Patient*
   A. To concentrate on quality, rather than quantity, of life.
   B. To allow the patient to die with dignity.
   C. To understand and care for the patient's physical, social, psychological, and spiritual needs (i.e., preserving the patient's integrity).
   D. To provide an environment for skilled nursing care (inpatient service).
   E. To provide rational relief of pain.

2. *Family Care*
   A. To provide support and education for the family, whether the patient is being cared for in the home or in the hospice.
   B. To understand and care for the family's physical, social, psychological, and spiritual needs (i.e., preserving the family's integrity).
   C. To provide 24-hour support and availability (the hot line).
   D. To use the same team that provides the inpatient service to support and educate the families and patients in their homes.
   E. To provide follow-up bereavement care for the family.

3. *Staff Care and Development and Consultation Service*
   A. To provide a model for maintaining the mental health and morale of health care staff serving the terminally ill.
   B. To provide a consultation service for other health professionals.

4. *Education*
   A. To provide a setting for education of health professionals in the care of the dying.

Patient Selection

The hospice (including inpatient, day, and home care) is designed for those patients with no longer any realistic hope of cure, for whom the prognosis of death is in a matter of weeks or months rather than years. It is not intended to be restricted to either geriatric or cancer patients. Patients may be of any age and may be suffering from cancer or nonmalignant conditions, such as multiple sclerosis or motor neuron disease. It may, however, be preferable for younger patients such as children or adolescents to be cared for in the main hospital where they can be with patients of the same age, and for the hospice team to participate in their care there. The patient must wish to come to the hospice, although this does not mean that they must know their own prognosis or even diagnosis. We would not wish to undermine a patient's defensive denial of illness.

To allow for home care the patient must live within easy traveling distance of the hospice. Since traveling time is more important than the number of miles traveled, we have set the limit at 30 minutes between the patient's home and the hospice. To provide home care, a "primary care person" in the home must be identified and it is this person who will be looking after the patient with the support of the hospice team. It is clearly not possible or desirable for the hospice team to assume direct 24-hour responsibility. The team will of course be available via the hot line.

The Patient Care Team

For each patient a team will be appointed that will have primary responsibility for the patient, both in the hospice and at home. The team will consist of a physician, a nurse, and one of the following: a social worker, psychologist, or counselor. There will also be close coordination with the unit receptionist, who is usually the first to be in contact with the family and the patient who is at home, and the housekeeper. Most health professionals with experience of inpatient care discover sooner or later that if they want to find out what a patient is really doing or feeling, the housekeeper or ward cleaner is a vital source of information. Many patients regard the housekeeper as someone they can easily relate to and who is "neutral" in their relationship with the health care team, as well as someone who can provide considerable support.

The Members of the Team

Members of the hospice staff will be employees of the larger hospital, but we hope that the staff will be functionally autonomous. A physician director will be appointed who will also be the leader of the team. It is essential to have a full-time hospice physician to provide necessary expertise for patient care. This person has not yet been identified.

It is important that the patient's own attending physician has input into patient management in order to provide continuity of care. But since the patient's own physician may not be skilled in palliative care, particularly in pain relief or providing necessary emotional support, we anticipate that much of the day-to-day management will be in the hands of the hospice physician. This bears a close parallel to other specialized units, such as intensive care units. The hospice team will be available for consultation elsewhere in the hospital.

The Hot Line

To provide necessary assistance, to foster self-confidence in patients and their families, and to support the primary care person in the home, there will be a telephone hot line. This will be a 24-hour service available for patients and relatives who are registered with the hospice. It will be an unlisted number and not given to anyone else. During regular hours, the receptionist will answer the call, determine if the caller needs a specific person, and act accordingly. The receptionist will transfer the call to the senior nurse on duty if no specific person is required. When no receptionist is on duty, the hot line will be answered at the nurse's station. Calls from the hospice will not be routed on the hot line to keep it as free as possible for emergencies.

Nursing Staff

We initially projected our nursing staff needs using the figure of 8.5 nursing hours per patient per day, a figure based on information from the Palliative Care Service at the Royal Victoria Hospital in Montreal (9). To provide nursing care at this level would be very expensive and we understand that the Montreal Palliative Care Unit (10) is now providing something in the order of 7.2 nursing hours per patient per day. The number of hours we finally provide will depend upon funds available. To provide the type of care we envisage will necessitate a high quality of nursing care, which is something that the committee felt was fundamental to the success of the unit. In addition to the nursing time for inpatient care, using information from active home care hospice programs, we will allow four full-time nurse equivalents for a predicted home care case load of 20.

Volunteers

Since this program, like most others, will be expensive, we will rely heavily on volunteers. There is an active group of volunteers working at St. John's Hospital but those who express a desire to help the hospice program will be specifically assigned to it. The volunteers will be able to perform various duties depending on each individual's particular skills and experience. In time it may be that individuals with personal hospice experience (those that have been bereaved) will volunteer to provide support for others suffering as they did (11).

Symptom Control

Based on the experiences of physicians who have prescribed the Brompton Mixture (two are on the Hospice Planning Committee) as well as information gathered from other units for the terminally ill, we developed the guidelines for pain control that we will use. Although heroin is not available in the United States, morphine is and an effective Brompton mixture can be prepared (12). Medical management of other symptoms will be in line with that reported by the Palliative Care Unit in Montreal (9).

Pain Control

The following elements of pain must be considered:

1. Physical
2. Mental

3. Financial
4. Interpersonal/Interfamilial
5. Spiritual

Aims of therapy to be used are:

1. Identification of etiology
2. Prevention of pain
3. Erasure of pain memory
4. To try to keep the patient functioning, alert, and aware of the surroundings as long as possible
5. Comfortable administration of medication (i.e., oral as long as possible)

Principles of therapy are:

1. Accurate diagnosis
2. Simple analgesics first
3. Narcotics when simple analgesics fail
4. Adequate dosage, titrated against the needs of the patient
5. Regular medication (not P.R.N.) to avoid (a) pain and (b) fear of pain
6. Remembering the patient and maintaining his or her integrity
7. Supporting the family
8. Utilizing other methods (e.g., palliative radiotherapy) when necessary
9. Remembering that, in terminal illness, drug addiction is not a hazard

Staff Support and Development

The development of the hospice unit will place stress on those working in it. This will be due not only to emotional pressures of caring for the dying and their families, but also to growth of the hospice as a new program. In an attempt to deal with the stresses, there will initially be weekly "bull and beef" sessions to allow staff to talk about their feelings. With luck these meetings can be transformed to more task-oriented management meetings before they become all "beef" and no "bull." We predict that the initial period of expansion will be particularly stressful. Careful selection of staff—avoiding particularly those individuals who are still resolving their own feelings about dying and death—will, we hope, be possible using careful interviewing and even psychological testing. We also plan a series of discussion groups to provide continuing education, considering topics such as pain relief, palliative nursing care, family dynamics, spiritual problems of the dying, etc. We feel that patients' interests will be best served by maintaining a task-oriented approach to patient care, while keeping personal staff support as a "hidden agenda" at staff meetings.

"Rules" of the Unit

Some of the rules that affect patients and visitors in nursing homes and acute medical beds are inappropriate for hospice patients. We intend to have visiting by relatives and friends of any age at any time of the day (possibly with a "rest day" once a week on the lines of St. Christopher's Hospice in London, which would allow relatives to catch up with washing, shopping, etc.). Patients will be encouraged to have their personal belongings around them. Social interaction and celebration of joyous occasions, such as birthdays, will be encouraged and the large room in the unit will be useful for this purpose. Visiting children will reinforce the feeling of life.

Medical Education within the Hospice

Education of future physicians is the key to improvement in the care of the dying in the community. We see the hospice as an invaluable opportunity to achieve the following objectives:

1. To educate medical students and residents in the care of the terminally ill in terms of palliative medical treatment, excellent pain control, family care, teamwork, and attention to detail in patient care and care of the "whole patient."
2. To expose medical students and residents to the hospice model in the care of the terminally ill.

    3. To demonstrate the possibilities of home care for the
       terminally ill.

Similar arrangements will be made for the education of other
health professionals. The close association between St. John's
Hospital and Southern Illinois University School of Medicine will
facilitate these goals.

Finance

Aside from the philosophical difficulties, the major stumbling
block to the development of programs for the terminally ill in
the United States has been that such programs are not generally
covered by Medicare, Medicaid, or health insurance companies.
It is likely that in due course hospice care will be supported by
a third party, but whether and when this happens will depend to
a significant extent upon impact of the hospices, such as ours,
developing throughout the United States.

    St. John's Hospital intends to go ahead with the unit and is
currently exploring the possibilities of obtaining start-up grants.
It is undesirable, for obvious reasons, for the program to be
dependent upon a grant of any sort and the unit hopes to be
self-supporting (or at least not losing too much money) by the
time any grant runs out.

Conclusion

The "nuts and bolts" of our plan as described may fail to
emphasize what is different about the hospice concept. The
emphasis of the program will be on care of the "whole"
patient—in terms of physical, social, psychological, spiritual, and
financial comfort.

    Francis Bacon wrote: "Men fear death, as children fear to go
in the dark; and as that natural fear in children is increased with
tales, so is the other." We hope that fear of the unknown may
diminish when patients and families see others dying without too
much suffering. We hope, too, that those who share in the
experience will themselves grow.

Our ideas are presently only on paper, so we are still blissfully unaware of most of our mistakes. However, the need for an alternative system of care of our terminally ill is clear, and even if some of the catch phrases have become somewhat hackneyed, we hope that the hospice will allow patients to "die with dignity."

References

1. Kübler-Ross, E. *On death and dying.* New York: Macmillan, 1969.
2. Saunders, C. *Care of the dying.* London: Macmillan, 1959.
3. Mount, B. M. The problem of caring for the dying in a general hospital; the palliative care unit as a possible solution. *Canadian Medical Association Journal,* 1976, *115,* 119–121.
4. Richardson, J. On dying and dying well. *Proceedings of the Royal Society of Medicine,* 1977, *70,* 71–73.
5. Dobihal, E. F. Talk or terminal care? *Connecticut Medicine,* 1974, *38,* 364–367.
6. Plant, J. Finding a home for hospice care in the United States. *Hospitals, Journal of the American Hospital Association,* 1977, *51,* 53–62.
7. Liegner, L. M. St. Christopher's Hospice, 1974. *Journal of the American Medical Association,* 1975, *234,* 1047–1048.
8. Kron, J. Designing a better place to die. *New York,* 1976, 43–49.
9. *Pilot Project Report Palliative Care Service.* Montreal, Royal Victoria Hospital, October 1976.
10. Ajemian, I., Personal communication 1977.
11. *News From Hospice.* New Haven, March 1975.
12. Mount, B. M., Ajemian, I., & Scott, J. F. Use of the Brompton Mixture in treating the chronic pain of malignant disease. *Canadian Medical Association Journal,* 1976, *115,* 122–124.

∞∞

PROBLEMS WHEN CARING

∞∞

ooo

THE EXPERIENCE OF AN ACADEMIC AS CARE GIVER: IMPLICATIONS FOR EDUCATION

ooooooooooooooooooooooooooooooooooooooooooooooooooooooooooooooooooooooooooooooooooooooo

Sr. M. SIMONE ROACH

Department of Nursing, St. Francis Xavier University
Nova Scotia, Canada

This article describes the experience of a nurse educator who participated in a 1-month course in the care of terminally ill and dying patients at St. Christopher's Hospice in London.

The writer, highlighting some features of this internationally known and respected model, discusses her personal reactions and the implications her experience could have for education. Emphasis is placed on the need for educators to become more aware of the demands—physical, emotional, and spiritual—which are made on those caring for terminally ill and dying patients, and of the unique personal needs that each care-giver may bring to this experience.

It is noted that not all persons who desire to care for terminally ill and dying patients necessarily have the capacity to do so, those who do require the assistance of a caring community.

Introduction

In June 1976, with the assistance of a World Health Organization Fellowship, I had the opportunity to participate in a 1-month course at St. Christopher's Hospice in London. This article is an attempt to describe the experience, the events leading up to it, and to share my personal response.

Much has been written about St. Christopher's by its own eminently qualified staff. Along with this contribution to the literature, Dr. Cicely Saunders, the founder-medical director, and members of the St. Christopher's team, have shared the fruits of their labors and research by lecturing at home and abroad, and by opening the doors of the hospice to international students and visitors.

My contribution would be redundant if it merely tried to tell the story of St. Christopher's, it would be pretentious and presumptuous if it claimed to report the contribution of St. Christopher's to individuals and groups seeking models for the care of terminally ill and dying persons. For such a story and report, I refer the reader to the already abundant literature, a list of which can be found in St. Christopher's library.

The following summary, which is St. Christopher's own description of its philosophy and orientation (1), will serve as background:

1. St. Christopher's is a Christian Foundation, ecumenical and practical, constantly searching for God's plan for its work and development.
2. It is a Medical Foundation, seeking to offer the best professional standards of care to patients with chronic and terminal pain, especially those with advanced malignant disease.
3. It is a community of people with a great diversity of experience and outlook who come together to welcome and help the whole family in the wards and in their own homes and after a patient's death.
4. Alongside a full commitment to the needs of each patient, it carries on research in clinical pharmacology, studying and evaluating drugs for the relief of pain and other terminal distress.
5. It is completing a series of psychosocial studies concerned with the problems and needs of mortally ill patients and their families and the help which can be offered to the bereaved.
6. It is a teaching hospice with a multidisciplinary programme concerned with developing understanding and skill in the whole field of the care of the dying.
7. It is a charity, founded and built entirely with gifts and grants and relying on them for a substantial part of its running costs.

8. It has firm links in policy and practice with the National Health Service, which currently supports its teaching and home care programmes as well as the maintenance of many of its patients.
9. St. Christopher's Hospice is open to all who need its care, regardless of race or creed or of their ability to pay anything towards the cost. Some wish to contribute towards the expenses of their care, and the remaining gap between government support and the full cost has so far been met mainly by the generosity of the Friends and other supporters of the Hospice. (p. 5)

An Overview of the Experience

After I arrived at the hospice, I found myself in a pleasant lounge in the Wates Study Center anxiously awaiting orientation. I was joined by three other equally anxious recruits. Two of these were a medical student and a social work student—both friendly and extremely warm persons. The third student was a young Episcopalian seminarian from Scotland who brought a rare combination of humor, mischief, depth, and commitment to our group. We were assigned to a tutor who, through the 4 weeks of our stay at St. Christopher's, shared generously of her expertise, but, most importantly, her personal gifts of warmth and human concern.

Looking back on the different backgrounds of this group of four—representative of medicine, nursing, social work, and theology—I wondered if the choice from the four disciplines was deliberate. At the time, our professional orientations did not seem important to us. What appeared to be important was what we had in common—an anxiety over what we had undertaken, a concern to learn all we could from the course, and, in the process of learning, to have a forum within which to share our interests and concerns. The relationship that developed became a significant factor in enabling us to cope with what at times became a very stressful experience.

It is also significant that, initially, our assignments were not based on the particular disciplines represented by each of us. We were assigned to wards to participate with staff in the care of patients. To enter into the care of persons during a critical phase of their "journey in life" was the task common to the four of us, regardless of our respective backgrounds or disciplines.

The program was organized to provide a balance of discussion sessions, review and critique of films, and experience on the wards. We were welcome to participate in all ward activities, including rounds, conferences, and social events. Library resources were made available to us, as were the comfortable facilities of the study center. One special highlight of the planned educational program was a weekly seminar with Dr. Colin Murray Parkes, social psychiatrist consultant to the hospice.

On the wards there was provision for expert physical care, and for individualized attention to each patient as a person. One of the jolting features of the ward environment, however, was the complete absence of equipment considered standard in the usual hospital setting. There were no thermometers, blood pressure machines, intravenous set-ups, oxygen masks, or monitors with which to become involved. This ward pattern of care called for a personal investment by all staff, without the support of gadgetry or technology.

The approach to pain control involved an effort to "destroy symptoms" while attempting to "preserve the person." The therapeutic regime established for each patient was to "anticipate" rather than "pursue the pain." That such a goal was being achieved was evident by the number of patients who, after being admitted in extreme distress and excrutiating pain, were, after a period of treatment, able to get out of bed, dress in their own clothes and, in some instances, walk around the grounds. Some patients became comfortable enough to return to their homes for awhile.

There was a radical openness toward the terminal nature of patients' diseased conditions and toward the reality of death. Neither were hidden nor denied. Nevertheless, patients' responses to these realities were quite varied. Patients were given the opportunity to prepare for and enter into the experience of a very important human event; the way this was done was conditioned by the resources of both patient and family. It was because of this philosophy of caring that the personal qualities of staff were so crucial. It was also because the reality of death was so visible that these same members of staff could be reminded daily of their own mortality.

The program had a strongly built-in community dimension. It was obvious that original plans for the physical facility placed a high priority on the value of providing for a community atmosphere. The hospice consisted of a 54-bed patient area, a 16-bed sitting room wing for elderly residents, and a day-care center for children of staff. The young and the old, those in the bloom of health and those with terminal illness, lived within the same complex. Death and dying were visibly part of the life continuum—death and dying were not isolated.

An important aspect of this community dimension was the responsibility assumed by staff to reach out to each family. Family members and friends of patients participated in the program of care and were made to feel at home in doing so. Visiting privileges were liberal. With the exception of a one day per week rest day for the family, there were no restrictions on visitors. However, even on this day family members stayed with patients if the situation so warranted. Through the follow-up care services of the domiciliary unit, some patients could be kept at home. In other situations, a patient may have been admitted only temporarily to allow the family a much needed respite before again resuming the care at home. Contact with the family continued after the patient died. In a real sense, the family was the "client."

On my first evening at St. Christopher's, I was privileged to participate in a unique community event—the monthly Pilgrim Club meeting. "Meeting" is hardly an appropriate label, for this get-together was more a friendly gathering of hospice staff relatives of patients who had died—people who socialized over a sherry or cup of coffee and seemed to enjoy just being there. I sat with a small group, one of whom seemed a "veteran" member, another a recently bereaved widow. It appeared to me that the atmosphere, the interest and caring approach of staff, and, most importantly, the presence of people who had experienced bereavement provided the kind of support that both the bereaved and the care givers needed.

Another aspect of the program that I believe enhanced the sense of community was the emphasis on spiritual care of patients, and the participation of staff in the spiritual dimension of hospice activities. The interdenominational chapel was the center of the physical structure and for many—patients, family, and staff—was very much the center of activity.

On my first morning on the ward I was informed that chapel services were being held, that patients who could and wished to attend were escorted there, and that staff were also free to participate. That morning I attended a very simple and beautiful prayer service conducted, not by the chaplain, but by the deputy medical director. This experience made real the assertion that prayer and praying, while neither imposed upon nor demanded of anyone, were the privilege and prerogative of all.

The deep faith, expressed in the philosophy of the hospice program, was articulated and visible in daily events and activities. Leading morning and evening prayers on the ward, attending to spiritual needs of patients, and carrying the prayer card were responsibilities as appropriate to the head nurse or staff nurse as were giving physical care or administering medications.

On the wards there was an atmosphere of freedom of religious expression, with no evidence of threat or embarrassment to those staff or patients who expressed no religious beliefs. For those with a personal faith, there seemed no need to preach or apologize. Being in tune with God was part of their lifestyle. They were simply expressing what was in their hearts.

A Personal Reaction

For a number of years, one of the obligations I considered myself to have as a nurse-educator was to provide some opportunity for health-related professional groups and other interested persons to deal with issues surrounding death and dying. Initially, my attention to this area resulted from recurring discussions about the unpreparedness of health professionals to respond to needs of dying patients, and the frequency with which related problems were treated in the literature.

This interest in terminal illness and death and dying is not, in itself, particularly significant. What is significant is the nature of peoples' reactions (myself included) to becoming involved in this particular area of study. These reactions ranged from a more academic interest and positive response indicating agreement that something needed to be done, to a more negative one, implying that such involvement suggested a preoccupation with death, or provided a way of dealing with one's own unresolved "loss" experiences.

I suspect that elements of both reactions motivated me to become involved in the study of death and dying and influenced my decision to go to St. Christopher's. Wherever I may stand on the above continuum—ranging from a purely academic interest to a preoccupation with and a searching for some way of dealing with personal experiences of death—the fact remains that, for whatever reason, it still seems very difficult in our society to talk about death and dying, to rationalize programs for study, to establish programs of care, and to decide how much of one's energy can be devoted to this area, academically and clinically.

My experience at St. Christopher's Hospice helped me to affirm what I had already accepted intellectually—that acceptance of life involves integrating the reality of death, and that dying well somehow includes the ability to enter consciously into and to achieve peace in that experience.

This affirmation came from the philosophy of care brought to life in practice on the wards, and by the lessons taught so well by the dying themselves. This affirmation came also from the nature of the complex, designed to provide for a community of persons in various stages of the life continuum in an environment where the rhythms of living and dying were seen as normal.

However enriching and affirming my experience at St. Christopher's was, it also became an increasingly difficult one. In retrospect, the difficulty could be simply labeled as "reality shock." This phenomenon, described by Kramer (2) in her study of a sampling of graduate nurses in the United States, relates to the conflicts arising out of a movement from a subculture that is familiar to a subculture that is not.

While reality shock, as described in the above study, is easy to understand as a phenomenon, and while, on reflection, it is not difficult to apply it to my experience at St. Christopher's, neither the nature of the conflict nor the elements of the conflict were clearly obvious to me while I was there. These elements are now discernible and include the following:

1. The role change from Canadian nurse educator and administrator to British nurse practitioner.
2. The unusualness of the hospice environment and its program of care.

It would seem I should have been able to address these conflict-causing factors as I experienced them. As I now perceive the situation, however, there was a further and perhaps a more fundamental conflict, namely, that the staff was there not for my benefit, but for the benefit of the hospice population. "I would not be 'professional' if I needed help!" "I was not supposed to have conflicts!"

The weekly seminar sessions with Dr. Colin Murray Parkes provided a rich opportunity for sharing the experiences we encountered on the wards. As a group, we related well and were at ease with Dr. Parkes because of his warmth, sensitivity, and nonthreatening manner. There was perhaps insufficient time to explore the more personal and deeper issues involved in our experiences.

During the next to last seminar with Dr. Parkes, the group began to get to some of these other issues, and I would have appreciated the opportunity to explore these further. However, I was still restrained by the feeling that it was not "appropriate" for me to reveal my personal reactions, not "appropriate" to seek a listening ear. I was there to learn not to be counseled. And this was my reaction, despite the fact that I believe that learning and counseling go together, and despite the fact that I believe that "professionals" also experience crises in their lives. At that time, all I would allow myself to do was to say, "Yes, I feel very sad."

The experience at St. Christopher's provided me with a great deal of knowledge and insight into what constitutes appropriate care for terminally ill and dying patients, but, as a person trying to learn and trying to care, trying to cope with problems which

I had not even allowed to surface, I was physically, emotionally, and spiritually drained. I survived because of the warmth and affirmation I received from the tutor, the group, and the few others at the hospice whom I got to know, and because of the opportunity provided by a friend to visit some of the beautiful and historical spots in England. I am sure that the time spent with the Lord, particularly in the daily Eucharist, was a source of great strength.

This experience has raised questions about the attributes necessary in those who care for terminally ill and dying patients, but it also raises further questions about the need to care for the care givers. With regard to the latter, I believe that caring is of one piece. Nevertheless, while we in the health field place much weight on *caring* as an essential component of practice, I do not believe that we have a very good record of either caring for ourselves of for each other.

St. Christopher's philosophy is that caring involves and needs a community of persons who support one another. There is no doubt that a spirit flowing from this philosophy enabled the initial core group to persist in making their dreams a reality, despite the many frustrations they encountered. I believe that the continuation of such a spirit and commitment to the vision of care promoted at St. Christopher's or elsewhere depend upon the preservation and/or development of a truly caring community.

Caring for persons with terminal illness and ministering to the dying is a difficult and sometimes painful mission, for the situation encountered can touch the core of one's being, where the urge to live and not to die is strong and unrelenting. Death is never beautiful. It says that something has gone wrong, that disharmony has taken over where harmony ought to have been. It symbolizes the epitome of broken and wounded humanity, in darkness and alone. According to Rahner (3) humanity is rightly afraid of death:

> Actually he should not die, for he still possesses within himself, that vitality of divine life, which if it could assert itself pure and unveiled in this earthly life, would completely eliminate death. (pp. 33–34)

The Christian believes that Jesus overcame death. But He overcame death by going through it. The death of Jesus was horrible, so horrible that all of nature seemed to bend under the strain. Rejoicing came only with the Resurrection three days later. While hope in the Resurrection dissipates despair, it does not right the wrong of the disharmony and disfigurement. Death remains the final unknown, the darkness through which every person must go before approaching the *light* in its fullness.

> The Christ who redeems us is the Christ *crucified*. The center of the Christian mystery, and therefore of the mystery of man, is the Cross. It was on the Cross that Christ brought forth from death to life: it is on the cross that the Christian, for his part, ceaselessly passes from life begun to life perfected, from life crucified to life re-arisen. (4, p. 134.)

What the care giver cannot do is remove the pain of death and separation. One cannot negate the cross. But the care giver can be present to share it and make its burden lighter. Even Jesus needed the presence of someone to help Him while His closest friends were terrified and fled.

There is nothing glamorous about caring for persons with terminal illness, and, as stated by one of the hospice staff (5), "living in a community whose business is the care of the very ill and of the dying is so hard that perhaps only a community can sustain it." Those for whom it is too difficult ought not to think that they are less generous or less humane. Their admission is an honest acknowledgement of the simple truth of human pain and limitation.

Our hope is bound up in faith, "for if we believe that Jesus died and rose, God will bring forth with him from the dead those also who have fallen asleep believing in him" (1Thes. 13:14. The New American Bible).

Implications for Education

My experience at St. Christopher's Hospice was rich in the opportunity it provided me to test out, in a real and unique setting, the ideas and expectations I had about the needs of terminally ill and dying patients, and about the nature and quality of services required to respond to these needs. Most important, it afforded me the opportunity to experience the kinds of demands made on the person practicing in this type of setting.

While there were uniquely personal factors in my background that shaped the nature and influenced the intensity of my response to the experience, I suspect that my overall reaction was not atypical. Because of this, and because of the experience of others with whom I worked in the setting, I believe that what I have shared in this overview has implications for how we work with learners, on any level, to enable them to care for terminally ill and dying patients. Some of the areas of conflict that I noted could have been experienced in any new setting. I believe others were conditioned by the nature of the setting itself.

I believe that educators need to become more aware of the demands—physical, emotional, and spiritual—which are made on those caring for terminally ill and dying patients, and of the unique personal needs each care giver may bring to this experience. This observation points to the responsibility of educators to prepare themselves and their students for the particular "subculture" of the practice setting, so different from that of classroom, workshop, or seminar, and indeed, because of the characteristics specific to the area of death and dying, which are different from other types of practice. I do not believe that educators can fulfill this responsibility without access to appropriate programs and settings.

One of the perennial frustrations of nurse educators is the difficulty in finding access to settings where what is believed in and taught is adequately modeled. This reality has caused, and continues to create, tension between a commitment to teach for *what is* or to teach for what *ought to be*. The program established at St. Christopher's Hospice, and in other models in the United States and Canada, give much hope that the tension can be lessened.

I believe that what is needed is not so much in providing new buildings or facilities, but rather in changing attitudes about what constitutes appropriate care for terminally ill and dying patients. I also believe that a small core of people, representative of the helping professions involved, and who are willing to commit themselves to this cause, can bring about the needed change. Educators can and ought to be part of this process.

Conclusion

On the basis of my reflections, I would conclude with the following observations applicable to both education and service:

1. If education truly means the development of persons, then educational programs ought to include some opportunity for teachers and students to reflect on the basic realities of human experience. Since one of these realities is death, some provision needs to be provided in a given curriculum to explore the theological, philosophical, and cultural dimensions of dying and death.
2. The opportunity to practice in a setting where appropriate care is modeled is a critical component of learning to care for terminally ill and dying patients.
3. Some provision for hypothetical models assists teachers and students in addressing themselves to issues and to come in touch with their own beliefs and feelings. While this is desirable and helpful, it does not necessarily anticipate the quality or the intensity of the reaction a person may have in the real situation.
4. In order to sustain a caring environment, and in order to enable care givers to use personal resources appropriately, measures need to be taken to provide a forum for discussion of personal reactions, and to assist them in assessing their capacity for this type of ministry.
5. Not all persons are able to cope with the demands of a setting for terminally ill and dying patients. For those who desire to do so, some type of human support system should be available, with training programs to provide guidance in the development and maintenance of support systems.

References

1. *St. Christopher's Hospice Annual Report 1974-1975*. London: St. Christopher's Hospice, 1976.
2. Kramer, M. *Reality shock: Why nurses leave nursing.* St. Louis: Mosby, 1974.
3. Rahner, K. *On the theology of death.* New York: Herder and Herder, 1961.
4. Mouroux, J. [*The meaning of man.*] (A. H. G. Downes, trans.). New York: Doubleday, 1971.
5. West, T. S. The final voyage. *Frontier,* 1974, *17*(4).

∞∞

MOTIVATION AND STRESS EXPERIENCED BY STAFF WORKING WITH THE TERMINALLY ILL

∞∞

M. L. S. VACHON

Clarke Institute of Psychiatry, and
University of Toronto, Ontario, Canada

Concern with needs of dying patients too often leads to neglect of corresponding needs of staff members who work with them. This paper describes how motivation of staff to work with dying patients can effect the job stress they encounter. It is suggested that staff often choose to work with the dying for one of six reasons: accident or convenience, a desire to do the "in thing" or to affiliate with a charismatic leader, intellectual appeal and a desire for mastery over pain and death, a sense of "calling," previous personal experience, and a suspicion that one might some day develop the disease.

Each motivation may lead to its own particular forms of stress. In addition, constant exposure to the dying can effect one's personal life and relationships with family members and friends. A number of suggestions are given for coping with job stress including: understanding one's own limits, maintaining a balanced personal life, and developing effective support systems on and off the job.

Introduction

All too often in our recent attempts to improve the care of the terminally ill we have negated and neglected the difficulties experienced by staff working with such patients. The metamessage is: "It's the patients who are sick and need help. We, the staff, are healthy and well-integrated and can cope cheerfully

An earlier version of this paper was presented at the International Seminar on Terminal Care, Montreal, P.Q, November 4, 1976.

with our daily exposure to disease, disfigurement and death. In fact, our very choice of a profession shows how healthy and competent we are."

Considerable experience with those who work with dying patients in a number of settings has caused the author to seriously question the above assumption. It is time to admit that many of us entered this field with hidden agendas and unmet needs. Our unacknowledged motivations can cause considerable stress and hinder relationships with patients, families, and other staff members. Much of this stress may be avoided if we take the time to look at the issues involved and learn to cope effectively with our own intrapersonal conflicts before they create unnecessary interpersonal difficulty.

In this paper the focus is off the dying patient and onto the needs of the professional in this field. The following areas will be explored:

1. Why we chose to work with dying patients.
2. How this motivation effects the stress we experience professionally.
3. What this work does to us personally.
4. What are the implications of the above and how we can improve our own coping mechanisms.

Why We Chose This Work

In discussing reasons behind one's decision to work with dying patients a clear distinction must be drawn between two groups: (1) those whose commitment is to patients with life-threatening illnesses, such as cancer, some of whom will live and some die, and (2) those whose major interest is care of the terminally ill where the goal is palliative care and a peaceful, hopefully meaningful, death. The experiences, frustrations and losses of these two groups are quite distinct as will become apparent in the following discussion of motivation and stress. Because of the nature of this volume, however, the present paper will focus primarily on needs of the latter group. The author has described some of the needs of the former group elsewhere (1-3).

In attempting to conceptualize reasons for working with dying patients, six major categories come fairly readily to mind although others, no doubt, might be equally valid and have their own inherent stress. The six major categories chosen are the following:

1. Accident, convenience, or a part of one's caseload.
2. A desire to do the "in thing" or to affiliate with a charismatic leader.
3. Intellectual appeal, that is, the desire for control and mastery over illness, pain, and death.
4. A sense of "calling" in religious or humanistic terms.
5. Previous personal experience either one's self or with those close to him or her.
6. The suspicion that one will someday develop the disease.

How Motivation Effects Stress

Occasionally an individual happens to be working with the terminally ill accidentally or simply for convenience. This probably occurs most often in a general hospital setting, where the assignment of nurses, social workers, and other professionals may be on the basis of unit need, rather than individual choice. Others may have found their way into settings such as oncology clinics through geographical proximity or a desire to work regular hours, rather than being motivated by any particular commitment to cancer patients.

This type of person can have a considerable advantage in such settings because while he or she may work quite hard, the position is regarded as simply a job. Personal involvement is minimized and the individual is not beset with ideas of failure if patients begin to deteriorate or die without reaching an idealized stage of acceptance.

If through proximity to dying patients, however, the person begins to become more emotionally involved than initially intended, problems may develop because the person's original concepts about the job have changed. With increased involvement comes increased risk. When one has not anticipated such involvement and perhaps even tried to avoid it, unexpected difficulty may result when certain patients with whom the individual is involved deteriorate or die.

Perhaps more often, the person who has come into this field by accident or through convenience will stay only so long as the job's rewards outweigh its hazards. If the going gets too rough, the individual will change jobs without too many qualms. Problems arise, however, when positions are scarce and a job transfer is not possible. In such situations, previously controlled stress escalates rapidly as one feels confined to a job where the emotional toll quickly becomes intolerable. Such people may then attempt to turn off all feelings and become quite cold or even hostile to patients.

If one is caring for dying patients as only a part of one's caseload, such as might happen with visiting nurses, the job stress of working with the dying may well be minimized as one goes from a patient who is doing well to one who is dying and perhaps finishes the day with a visit to a new mother. In such instances death is seen in its proper perspective—as another part of life. Frustrations may arise, however, because a lack of expertise may cause the individual to feel impotent and isolated when dealing with severe problems with pain, nausea, weakness, constipation, and fear so common in the dying person. In addition, peer support and outside consultation may be unavailable in such community settings.

The second motivation for choosing to work with the dying is a desire to do the "in thing" or to affiliate with a charismatic leader. As the field of thanatology becomes increasingly popular, many people are becoming fascinated by the idea of working with the dying. For some it has become yet another bandwagon to join. Such individuals may have been "converted" by listening to one of the charismatic leaders in the field, through reading the extensive literature, or through a growing personal awareness of the problems confronting the dying. Often staff members may be attracted to particular settings by the presence of charismatic leaders. They anticipate considerable exposure to such authorities and expect to develop an intense relationship with the expert, which will serve to nourish and sustain the neophyte both personally and professionally.

Frequently with this type of motivation the glamor of working with dying patients wears thin as one discovers that they are not all young, beautiful, and articulate people who are longing to spend their dying months talking about their philosophy of life and death. Instead they may well be quite sick with distasteful physical symptoms, impatient with talk, and want to deny the fact that they are dying.

The charismatic leaders who were expected to function as role models and mentors may be out on lecture tours and talking to important visitors much of the time. Even when present, they may prove to be all too human as their theories and charisma may not always work in this field where no one has all the answers. The individual who has chosen to blindly follow a charismatic leader may become very frustrated and angry in such situations. Often the cause of these emotions is unrecognized because one must not think ill of the leader, as it was once thought one must not speak ill of the dead. Instead, tension escalates and is projected onto other staff members, often those given authority in the leader's absence. As tension among staff members increases, patient care may deteriorate until such time as the operative process is identified. In such situations, those attracted because of the expected glamor of the job may leave and the others begin the process of "de-throning" the leader and coming to develop more realistic expectations of this individual and of their own role within the setting.

The third reason for entering the field of thanatology is intellectual appeal, that is, a desire to gain control and mastery over illness, pain, and death. Such an individual may make a significant scientific contribution, but may arouse considerable hostility from colleagues who may see attempts to quantify pain relief, illness stages, methods of intervention with the dying, etc., as intrusive and threatening to undermine the staff member's control, skills, and role.

Scientific investigation is needed in this field, but those whose primary commitment is research must be warned that they will usually be ambivalently regarded both by the staff who work with the dying as well as by peers in the scientific community. Furthermore, if the scientist at an unconscious level is really attempting to gain control and mastery over these issues of life and death, constant exposure to the realities of pain and suffering may lead to a breakdown in normal defense patterns, particularly intellectualization. Significant depression may ensue, especially if the researcher has now begun to become emotionally aware of, and involved in the suffering of the dying.

The fourth motivation in caring for the dying is a sense of "calling" in religious or humanistic terms. This type of motivation can augur well for working in thanatology because of the dedication it implies but it may also prove to be problematic. Such people tend to become quite involved with patients and they approach the job with missionary zeal. No demand is too great. They are on call 24 hours a day, 7 days a week. Such involvement can lead to depletion, however, unless one has some outside source of replenishment—spiritual, interpersonal, or both.

Although it is often argued, and rightfully so, that working with the dying has its own rewards, one cannot expect all one's satisfaction to come from one's patients. First of all, it places an unfair burden on patients to meet the unmet needs of staff. Second, it leaves the staff member open to considerable loss each time a patient dies. Staff working with the dying need to have friends and support systems among the living as well as among the dying.

Another problem confronted by those who enter this field because of a sense of calling is the difficulty others have when exposed to a surfeit of virtue. They may admire such dedication but it may also make them feel guilty and useless, as well as hostile and resentful. Patients also may feel guilty and be unable to speak of their lack of religious faith or past sins to a person who seems unable to understand certain aspects of people's humanity. On a more practical level, sometimes such people seem so "other worldly" that mundane matters such as wet beds go unnoticed and others are afraid to mention such problems to them.

The fifth motivation is previous personal experience, either one's own self or that of a close relative or friend. This type of motivation is admirable and often such people have considerable insight to offer. However, it is important to note that insofar as possible, previously unresolved grief experiences should be worked through before one begins to work with the dying. Otherwise one might be motivated primarily by guilt and/or a desire to prove to be better than those who cared for the individual or relative. When the past is unresolved the person may rapidly become depleted because of trying to accomplish too many jobs at once. In addition, problems of overidentification with those patients who remind the person of the past prove to be a problem not only for the individual but also for fellow staff members working with the same patient. Peculiar power struggles may develop as staff members overidentify with particular patients and project incompetence onto one another.

The final motivating factor is the suspicion that one day the individual will develop the disease. People with a personal or family history of a particular disease may well be attracted to working with patients with the disease as well as those who are dying of it. This attraction may occur for a number of reasons, including a desire for knowledge of the disease and personal access to those who treat it, a need to give to others now so that one will be thought to be deserving of special care later, and an attempt to give to others what one is certain no one could give to him or her. This motivation and the involvement that ensues may cause friction and isolation from colleagues who cannot quite understand the underlying dynamics of the situation but know only that this particular staff member seems to have an inordinate need to be needed.

In addition, there may be an overidentification with particular patients that may lead to the isolation of both the staff member and the patient. Finally, such a person may feel more threatened than other staff members when several patients die in quick succession or when a particular patient with whom there was strong identification dies.

What This Work Does to Us Personally

Given that many of us have entered the field of thanatology with greater or lesser degrees of unconscious or subconscious motivation that we can hopefully resolve, how else does our choice of profession affect us? One does not have to be in the field too long to begin to feel the stigma it entails. At a social gathering any mention of one's profession may bring a most peculiar form of attraction/repulsion. Even families may regard this type of job with more than the usual degree of ambivalence and may urge a job change, refuse to allow any discussion of death at home, or complain vehemently at the intrusion that involvement with dying patients can make on one's home life.

Not only are our families threatened by work with the dying, but for us too, the work can be quite threatening at times. While one might derive a certain unacknowledged feeling of omnipotence in walking through the valley of death knowing it's not yet his or her turn, it must be acknowledged that someone working in thanatology may eventually come to feel surrounded by death and succumb to depression and the helpless/hopeless attitude that can predispose us to our own illnesses. Still another response to the omnipresence of death is acting out behavior on the part of staff members almost as an affirmation of life. Such behavior can occur in many way, perhaps the most common being sexual acting out, excessive drinking, or taking unnecessary risks such as speeding.

Finally, there is the problem that results when the thanatologist's family member is sick or dying. This often causes role confusion because, on the one hand, the person is supposed to be an expert on death and, on the other hand, feels perhaps even more impotent than others in facing impending death in a relative. After all, what can "experts" say to a close relative facing death. The expert role may well get in the way of the personal relationship.

Implications and Ways to Improve our Coping

What then are the implications? Most important is the acknowledgment that the staff member who works in thanatology is first and foremost a person who has needs, motivations, and stress. While we cannot rightfully expect hospice units to act as therapeutic milieus for the staff, it is possible to set forth some basic principles:

1. Individual staff members should be encouraged to gain personal insight so as to understand and acknowledge their own limits. It should be acknowledged that one's limits vary over time and extra support or time off may have to be provided when staff members are under a high degree of stress. However, the needs of patients do deserve top priority and if certain staff members constantly require considerable support they should be encouraged to seek employment elsewhere.

2. A healthy balance must be maintained between work and an outside life. While this type of work demands considerable personal involvement and cannot realistically be a 40-hour-a-week job, there must be times when staff are totally off-call and left to pursue their own life-affirming activities.

3. The individual must be careful when the "need to be needed" becomes too great and he or she attempts to be everything to everyone. This work is probably best accomplished by a team. Although many in the field are strong individualists, a team approach to much of the work is crucial.

4. The individual must maintain a support system at work and outside the work setting. Hospice units must make some provision for ongoing staff support through the use of visiting psychiatric consultants for the staff, weekly staff support meetings or other models that seem appropriate to a given unit. In addition, individuals should be encouraged to seek relationships outside the work setting for additional support. All too often staff members working in hospice settings become a closed social network, isolating themselves from friendships with others outside the field.

5. For those working in isolation, it may be wise to seriously consider ongoing contact with an outside consultant and/or therapist who can offer guidance as needed and provide much needed support as well.

Conclusion

In conclusion, it has been shown that the conscious and unconscious factors that motivate individuals to work in thanatology may well lead to unexpected stress. This stress can pose significant problems for patients and other staff members with whom we work. In addition, job stress can carry over into one's personal life causing individual and family problems.

The reader may feel that the author's comments are too negative and that she has failed to acknowledge "pure" motivation some thanatologists may have. The author apologizes for any such oversights and reiterates that the paper's purpose is to point up some of the problems staff members may have in this field. The author certainly does not contend that all staff members are laboring under tremendous unconscious needs, rather that many of us have entered the field with some unmet needs and unacknowledged motivations that may lead to later difficulty. If we can develop insight into our own needs and provide effective staff support systems, then the high level of patient care found in most hospice settings will be maintained at minimal psychic cost to staff members.

References

1. Vachon, M. L. S. Enforced proximity to stress in the client environment. *Canadian Nurse,* 1976, *72*(9), 40-43.
2. Vachon, M. L. S., Lyall, W. A. L., & Rogers, J. The nurse in thanatology: What she can learn from the womens' liberation movement. In A. M. Earle, N. T. Argondizzo, & A. H. Kutscher (Eds.), *The nurse as caregiver for the terminal patient and his family.* New York: Columbia University Press, 1976.
3. Vachon, M. L. S., Lyall, W. A. L., & Freeman, S. J. J. Measurement and management of stress in health professionals working with advanced cancer patients. *Death Education,* 1978, *1*, 365-375.

Request reprints from M. L. S. Vachon, Community Resources Section, Clarke Institute of Psychiatry, 250 College St., Toronto, Ontario, Canada M5T 1R8.

∞∞∞

USING THE CREATIVE PROCESS
WITH THE TERMINALLY ILL

∞∞∞

BARRY LeGROVE ROGERS
Hillhaven Hospice, Tucson, Arizona

Problems faced by terminally ill patients and the ways those problems are addressed by institutional care givers may thwart the patient's creative impulses, which are basic to living. This essay describes how the staff of Hillhaven Hospice encourages and supports the creativity of patients through the medium of creative writing.

It is my belief that the arts are at the center of learning in the development of the whole person and that the quality of life is dependent on acknowledgement and acceptance of creativity as part of daily living.

The creative process is the distillation of energy, the concentrated essence of the life process. It is widely accepted that much of great art is produced under stress, out of frustration, as an expression of anxiety, or as a result of intense need to communicate. The creative process is often stifled for many people and, under stress, the energy level builds rapidly and with it the need to express. However, most people do not have methods or techniques available for harnessing these energies into a positive and productive outlet. When a person confronts death, perhaps the time of greatest stress in one's life, the arts become a valuable tool both to inspire and to serve as a medium in which to express innermost thoughts, fears, and expectancies.

There is growing interest and much research into possible correlation between psychological stress factors and emergence of cancer cells (1, 2). If in the future a greater emphasis is placed on an acceptance of the arts as an ordinary element of living, if to write a poem or to paint a picture is as normal as eating breakfast, then possibly we can reverse the terrible increase in the incidence of cancer. Of course, we must continue the research into pollution of the air we breathe and the food we eat.

Our aim at the hospice is to provide as many artistic stimuli as possible in the form of performance (music, dance, drama) and presentation (movies, slide shows), and to create a relaxed atmosphere (birthday and cocktail parties) in which the creative process can be released as a normal and acceptable part of living. Let us remind ourselves constantly that living, as a normal functioning and productive state of being, should continue up to the moment of death.

Whenever possible, within a few days of admission the patient at Hillhaven is taken for a tour of the hospice and grounds in a golf cart to help with orientation. In many medical facilities, patients are whisked immediately to their rooms on arrival, often on stretchers, which disorients them to their environment.

At Hillhaven, patients share their ride with another patient. A meeting follows with more patients in a nonthreatening environment with perhaps a glass of wine and a slide presentation to keep attention away from the individual.

All patients are evaluated by personal interview under four general headings:

1. Current level of functioning (mental and physical)
2. Likes and dislikes
3. Hopes and fears
4. Experiences and expectations

Interviews are carried out in a relaxed conversational atmosphere and an attempt is made to establish a point of relationship, a mutual understanding and acceptance, and an emphasis on the matter of choice by patients as to the focus of their energies. Butler and Lewis (3) have been referred to in creating guidelines for diagnostic evaluation but the completion of data forms, either by patients or by the Director of Creative Communications in their presence, is avoided so patients will not feel as though they are under some form of analysis.

Implementation of the creative communications philosophy is supported by the occupational therapist and the rest of the team involved in a counseling situation in order to achieve a spiritual and emotional balance for patients and their families. This team, consisting of the social worker, the chaplain, the occupational therapist, and the director of creative communications, works together, overlapping their energies, varied skills, and personalities to reach this balance.

Many crafts and art media are available as outlets for creative energy but those with quick results are particularly useful (Ojo de Dias—Gods Eyes—takes a few minutes to learn and in an hour can produce quite spectacular results). It is important that new skills be chosen for their simplicity and short-term effect. We look for outlets for creative energy and work for achieving serenity and peace of mind.

Because many cancer patients, due to illness or age, have deteriorating physical capacities (edema, arthritis, failing vision, general debility), a great deal of emphasis is placed on creative writing—which can be accomplished by tape recording or by dictating to an individual as well as by the physical act of writing. Thus, more patients can engage in creative writing than any other art medium, which is fortunate because through writing, one can have not only a creative outlet but also means to achieve other advantages in the form of putting one's life in perspective. Thus, major emphasis is placed on encouraging reminiscence and journal writing.

Progoff (4) is a highly recommended introduction to this field. Writing as a form of nonthreatening therapy (no judgments or diagnoses are made) helps people examine their lives, become aware of achievements, come to terms with guilt feelings and inadequacies, and, therefore, deal with the uncertain time of transition they now face. A journal, whether written or recorded, is also a fine legacy to pass to their families, communicating feelings of love and appreciation to loved ones.

Poetry writing is also encouraged through regular workshops in which poetry is taught as an art and not as some form of therapy. "As therapy it may help someone to be a busy old person but as art and accomplishment it can help him to be fully alive" (5). The advantage of poetry is that accuracy of detail and chronology are unimportant. Poetry is a way of expressing the essence of an emotion in a concise and precise way, whereas with prose a person is more inclined to ramble. As soon as people understand that poetry does not have to have a set meter and rhyme and that a natural rhythm will grow out of the content, they can be guided easily through a poetic expression of their emotions. Poetry writing has been particularly useful in helping family members remember the patient at the high point of his active life before the illness.

A newsletter has been established at Hillhaven Hospice to share thoughts, exchange ideas, and most of all to set a stage for the products of creativity.

We are working to further develop this theory of the value of the creative process for persons moving through an uncertain time of transition. Our work will continue to explore all areas of creativity—as an inspiration to a quality of life and as an outlet for energies toward the achievement of balance of mind and emotional and spiritual serenity.

References

1. Bronner, H. J. The psychological aspects of cancer in man. *Psychomatics*, 1971, *12*(2), 133-138.
2. Gussom, J. J. Psychological correlates of cancer. *Journal of Consulting Clinical Psychologists*, 1975, *43*(1), 113.
3. Butler, R. N., & Lewis, M. I. *Aging and mental health.* St. Louis: Mosby, 1977.
4. Progoff, I. *At a journal workshop.* New York: Dialogue House, 1977.
5. Koch, K. *I never told anybody.* New York: Random House, 1977.

ꝏꝏ

A GUIDE TO EVALUATION RESEARCH IN
TERMINAL CARE PROGRAMS

ꝏꝏ

ROBERT W. BUCKINGHAM III and SUSAN H. FOLEY
Columbia University, New York

Pressure for greater accountability is being exerted on programs for care of the terminally ill and increasing the demand for evaluation research. Current documentation of such programs is inadequate in that it is anecdotal and consists primarily of conjecture and case studies fraught with unsubstantiated value judgments. Information essential to the improvement of such programs and the determination of their effectiveness can be derived only through the application of strict experimental methodology. The components, implications, and limitations of rigorous evaluation systems are discussed, and their application in the terminal care setting addressed. The Buckingham evaluation of a hospice's home care service is cited as the first attempt at measurement of the overall quality and effectiveness of a hospice program, and as a model for future evaluation of similar hospice programs.

Health care research is often casually equated with research in biology and symbolized by the figure of a white-coated laboratory scientist bending over a microscope, absorbed in the empirical evidence emanating from a drop from a test tube. Such a narrow perspective of health care research neglects evaluative research designed to address the issue of quality of care as perceived by the consumer of that health care service.

Scientific research can be divided into three categories: (1) basic research that extends the scope of science and effects its general laws, (2) developmental research that produces techniques for the application of existing knowledge, and (3) applied research that provides knowledge needed to accomplish a particular goal. None of the three types can be considered more necessary than another in terms of human benefit; indeed, the divisions are subject to much dispute. Seen as a continuum, basic knowledge is required for the broadening of the substantive potential of science whereas applied science is essential to the realization of that potential.

It is my belief that the most urgent need in the field of terminal care is the need for applied research and development— the extension of basic knowledge of the needs of the dying and the determination of the best way to meet those needs through the use of biomedical and social science methodology.

Increasing demands for greater accountability are currently affecting the field of terminal care. Despite the emergence of a somewhat consistent philosophy of terminal care, the greatest portion of the literature on death and dying is theoretical and anecdotal. The lack of substantiating evidence in support of presently operative theories, the obvious need for better care, and the pending support of many service facilities all call for documentation to replace the overabundance of conjecture and opinion in the field of death and dying with a solid foundation on which to base action programs. The process of forming judgments regarding worth of a program for care of the terminally ill must utilize procedures designated for collection and analysis of data that increase ability of proponents to prove rather than merely claim the value and effectiveness of that program.

In order to justify continuation as well as the proposed extension of the hospice concept, proof of program legitimacy and effectiveness is required. As investments in terms of professional training and community resources develop around the specialized area of terminal care, demand for proof of the validity of services will continue to increase. Determination of the extent to which current hospice programs are meeting the challenges they address is essential to improvement of the functioning of such programs in the presence of social and administrative limitations. Solutions to problems in caring for the terminally ill can be most effectively obtained through planned action based on existing knowledge, and gradual improvement based on the discovery and accretion of new knowledge.

If new knowledge is to be incorporated into an established program, an evaluation of ongoing activities must be carried out to determine the best reallocation of resources, and prior testing of proposed activities must be accepted as a prerequisite to their practical implementation. However, valid interpretation and fruitful application of research findings seldom takes place. Personal and experiential bias prevent the dedicated health care worker from realizing that the need for programs of terminal care does not guarantee the effectiveness of solutions proposed to meet that need. Thus, future progress in the field of terminal care will be contingent upon the implementation of valid and reliable research data as well as its accumulation.

Evaluative research refers to measurement of consequences of interventions imposed to further a valued goal. Such research relies on scientific methods for examining effectiveness of planned changes. Because evaluation facilitates progressive adjustment toward attainment of a goal, it can and should play a key role in program planning and development. The aim of evaluative research extends beyond the determination of success or failure toward ascertaining why success or failure occurred and what actions can and should be taken. The role of program evaluation in perfecting policies and interventions is illustrated in Figure 1.

Use of the scientific method in performing such an evaluation requires considerable forethought as well as scrupulous attention to detail. Before an evaluation can take place, goals of the health care program must be identified and translated into measurable terms. Precognition of the problems with which the program must cope is advised lest the exigencies of program development invalidate an ongoing, inflexible course of evaluation. Program activities should be profiled and standardized to facilitate measurement of changes that take place. Measures used to monitor effectiveness of program activities should have proven reliability and validity. Where changes are detected, the possibility that they may be due to some factor other than the activity of the program should be considered. Those effects attributable to work of the program should be rated for durability and generalizability. Progress in evaluation of terminal services will be made as a function of use of the scientific

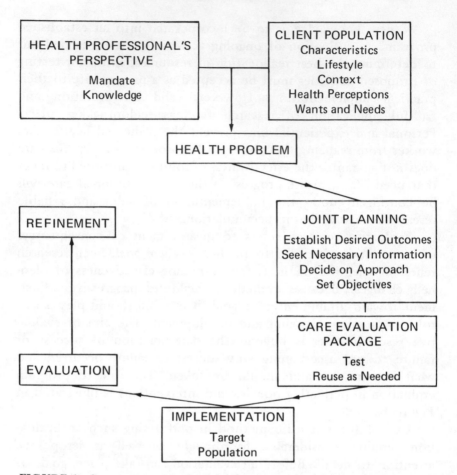

FIGURE 1 Consumer-centered model for program evaluation.

method—the examination of program objectives and their atten-
dant assumptions, the development of measurable criteria expli-
citly related to those objectives, and controlled determination of
the extent to which the objectives are met characterize true
evaluative research as distinct from subjective assessment. An
evaluation of a hospice home care facility can accomplish even
more than discovery of whether and to what extent objectives
have been met. An evaluation can pinpoint causes of specific
successes and failures and direct program planners toward formu-
las of success. An initial evaluation can provide a framework for
subsequent investigation and allow anticipation of success from

previously assessed interventions. Goals can be made operational and even redefined on the basis of preliminary findings. However, because evaluation is so closely related to program planning and operation, the potential for conflict between administrative and research interests is inherent in the evaluation process.

Practical problems of adhering to principles of research, in opposition to administrative considerations, constitute a greater challenge to execution of an evaluative study than do the rigors of those principles. Principles of research dictate that specific activities should be measured rather than entire programs, that methods and objectives of terminal care programs should be clearly defined, and that control groups as a basis for comparison should be used. However, the nature of most social service programs works against application of experimental methodology. Service personnel, although highly qualified for delivery of terminal care, usually have neither the training nor the skills necessary for evaluative research. The collection and interpretation of data are unsophisticated as a consequence and suffer from the lack of strict scientific guidance. Furthermore, the irregularity with which scientific standards are adhered to by various staff members results in collection of unreliable data. Attempted self-evaluation by terminal care programs not only incorporates problems of ill-prepared personnel, but also inevitably precludes objectivity. Personal bias is unavoidable when funding or reputation of one's program is at stake. In addition, the need to carry out self-evaluation as well as usual service activities prevents allocation of sufficient time, money and personnel for planning, collection of data, and analysis. Unfortunately, administrative resistance and barriers, lack of resources and failure to utilize findings frequently operate against objective evaluation, which is the preferable alternative to self-evaluation.

In the event of administrative cooperation, the subject matter may pose problems for evaluation of facilities for terminal care. Arbitrary selection of target problems stresses traditional activities at the expense of developing areas. Evaluation of facilities and resources is frequently emphasized while effectiveness of interventions is ignored. The Donabedian model of evaluative research (1), utilized in evaluation of home care services at Hospice, Inc., in New Haven, proposes an appealing

solution to substitution of facilities and activities for achievement. Donabedian perceives resources and effort expended as
matters of importance in characterization of the program rather
than the assessment of program effectiveness. He has outlined a
structure for evaluation that points to three components—
structure, process, and outcome—as the basis for evaluation. It is
measurement of outcomes that allows determination of program
effectiveness, and description of structure and process that
provides the basis for assumptions of causality. Program goals
and objectives are the dependent variables of such an evaluation.

The problems, objectives, and methods involved in application of a scientific evaluative design can be most thoroughly
understood via examination of a specific application. The outcome evaluation of home care services provided in New Haven is
not only a clear example, it is the only study of its kind that
has been carried out in a hospice setting (2). The long-term goal
of this project has been to evaluate the hospice home care
program. An appraisal of end results or outcomes has been used
in assessing the quality of care received by patients and families
under the program. In gauging the influence of elements comprising the hospice approach to terminal care, physical symptoms (e.g., subjective complaints such as pain, weakness, anxiety,
or depression caused by biological abnormalities), psychological
symptoms (e.g., subjective complaints generated by emotional
problems), and functioning of patient and family as individuals,
family members, and members of society were the foci of major
concern.

The objective of the evaluation has been to determine
whether hospice staff has been meeting its stated goal of
lowering levels of anxiety and depression experienced by
patients and their primary care persons. To accomplish this
objective, the home care milieu has been evaluated. Since the
intensity of perceived anxiety and depression are determined by
both physical and psychological processes, the hospice approach
to maintenance of patient/family well-being encompasses treatment of many vectors contributing to the experience of negative
affect. It has been the goal of the evaluation of services at the
hospice in New Haven to determine whether the hospice program of terminal care, by providing for many needs that often

cannot be met in acute care settings, is in fact more successful at relieving these symptoms among its patients and primary care persons than other facilities attending to the terminally ill.

In order to find evidence for or against the thesis that the hospice home care program provides effective care to its terminal patients, the director of evaluation chose to compare anxiety, depression, and social adjustment scores of a hospice and a nonhospice patient/family group as obtained from the Symptom Checklist 90 (3), Social Adjustment Self-Report (4), and Zuckerman Adjective Checklist (5) instruments. The hospice patient/family group consisted of all breast, lung, and colon cancer patients and their primary care persons who enrolled in the home care program during the study period of September 1, 1975 to May 31, 1977, and met the study criterion of 14 days survival after introduction of hospice services. The nonhospice patient/family control group was selected from outside the hospice geographical service area on referral of the same physicians who referred hospice patients. To reduce extraneous influences of age, sex, and primary site on any subsequent analysis, samples were similarly stratified with respect to each of these variables: individuals chosen for the control group were selected to approximate age, sex, and disease site characteristics of members of the hospice group. This purposeful categorization qualified the total grouping of hospice and control patient-primary care person subjects as a stratified convenience sample.

The hospice and control groups differed with respect to the spectrum of treatment modalities they received in accordance with differing therapeutic philosophies of organizations charged with their care.

Indices of anxiety, depression, and social adjustment were derived from the three self-report questionnaires used in the study. The self-report mode of psychological measurement was selected for its many advantages. Self-report provides access to information that is unobtainable through other channels: responses obtained are those of the experiencing individual, not an objective clinical observer whose report, however insightful, is limited to verbal and behavioral manifestations of affect. Although question bias may remain undetected, self-report measures can eliminate the danger of interviewer bias and economize administrative and scoring time. In addition, probe questions are not required, and avoidance of missing data can be maximized if a trained representative monitors completion of the questionnaire.

The specific aim of this paper was to ascertain whether the hospice home care program is meeting its specific goals by testing the following hypotheses:

1. Hospice patients exhibit lower levels of anxiety and depression as measured by the Zuckerman, Lubin, and Symptom Checklist 90 scales than the nonhospice comparison group.
2. Hospice patients exhibit higher levels of social adjustment as measured by the Social Adjustment Self Report Questionnaire than the nonhospice comparison group.
3. Hospice primary care persons exhibit lower levels of anxiety and depression as measured by the Zuckerman and Lubin and Symptom Checklist 90 than the nonhospice comparison group.
4. Hospice primary care persons exhibit higher levels of social adjustment as measured by the Social Adjustment Self Report Questionnaire than do the comparison nonhospice group.

Such explicit delineation of evaluation objectives is vital to proper execution of a rigorous evaluative study, and requires collaboration of research and administrative personnel. Methods suitable to measurement of stated program goals include use of an appropriate research design, selection of a representative (preferably randomized) sample, and use of valid and reliable instruments for collection of data.

A static-group comparison was chosen in which a group that experienced services of the hospice home care program was compared with a group that did not, for the purpose of establishing the effect of those services. The design was an equivalent group post-test design and was employed to establish the effect of the home care program by facilitating a comparison of outcomes (6, p. 12).

Familiarity with the nature of the hospice program was

necessary for selection of a sample from that population. All patients who enroll in the hospice program enter during the terminal stages of cancer, with a clinical prognosis of 6 months or less. Of this total population, over 50 percent have cancer with a primary site of either lung, colon, or breast. The questionnaire was administered throughout the 2-year study period to all patients with these diagnoses who survived the program more than 2 weeks, constituting a total sample size of 35 patients receiving hospice care. The three designated primary sites were specified as criteria for admittance into the study in order to facilitate the acquisition of a matched control.

The comparative sample consisted of patients who met all criteria for acceptance into the hospice program except one: they did not reside within the hospice geographical area. They were similar to hospice patients with respect to other qualifications for admission. Members of both groups had a confirmed diagnosis of terminal cancer with a projected survival time of 6 months or less, had lived with a friend or relative with the potential for functioning in the role of primary care person, were no younger than 18 years, and had been referred by the same oncologists as refer the hospice population in general.

The total number of patients comprising the control sample was 35. These patients were matched with the hospice group with respect to age (within 10 years), sex, and primary site of cancer.

Collection of information on the background and stable characteristics of hospice and nonhospice patients and primary care persons was required to ensure comparability of psychosocial scores. Random selection of subjects—the ideal method for achieving maximum comparability of groups—was not feasible due to time limitations and small population size.

Demographic data regarding age, sex, education, occupation and financial circumstances were obtained from existing records, from specific items requested in a portion of the self-report questionnaire sequence, and from the hospice routine data retrieval system. Subcultural information concerning ethnicity, religion, and religiosity was gathered in the same manner. The history of the patient's terminal illness, prognosis, major medical complications, and the patient's awareness of the illness has been cataloged by means of the data retrieval system.

Demographic and subcultural data similar to that collected on hospice patients were compiled in the same manner for hospice primary care persons. The relationship of the primary care person to the patient was also noted.

Demographic data regarding age, sex, education, occupation, and financial circumstances, and subcultural information concerning ethnicity, religion, and religiosity were obtained for patients in the comparison group from questionnaire items, routine forms and records kept by the primary physician. This information, along with the history of the patient's terminal illness, was extracted from the medical records with consent of the primary physicians.

Documentation that the hospice and control groups were similar on variables relevant to comparison was basic to the final analysis of outcomes. Characterization of the consumers of home care was thus carried out in conjunction with precise measurement of outcomes to ensure comparability of service group results on anxiety and depression scores. Choice of statistical tests to be used in the comparison of mean values of variables measuring anxiety, depression, and social adjustment was contingent upon assumptions that could be made regarding demographic distribution of hospice and nonhospice groups. Findings of the evaluation of hospice home care services in New Haven indicate that hospice patients and primary care persons exhibited higher levels of social adjustment and lower levels of anxiety and depression than nonhospice patients and primary care persons. However, interpretation of these results must be tempered by an awareness of circumstances and problems involved in conducting such a study with terminally ill patients.

It is estimated that nonhospice patients spent 50 percent more time in either an acute care hospital or some other form of institutional setting than hospice patients. Nonhospice patients were channelled in and out of hospitals to a greater extent than were hospice patients, and, as a consequence, spent less time living with their families. Few patients in the nonhospice study group received any form of home care service. A strong possibility exists, therefore, that home care and not hospice service as such was the critical element in alleviating problems of terminal illness for hospice patients and their families. However, if this is true, the fact remains that Hospice, Inc., has presented itself as an effective vehicle for such home care assistance. Further study is called for to determine which elements of hospice care are specifically responsible for improvements detected in the hospice group.

As is the case with any study attempting to evaluate a federally funded service program, gratitude of patients and primary care persons receiving free care and their unwillingness to seem critical of such care are potential sources of study bias. Introduction of fee-for-service hospices with compatible evaluation programs might eventually solve this problem.

According to subjective assessment of the interviewer, non-hospice patients experienced more pain than hospice patients. It is rational to assume that prolonged terminal suffering tends to sap the vital energy of an individual that would otherwise be utilized in coping with tremendous emotional, spiritual, and practical burdens of dying. The possibility exists, therefore, that application of the hospice philosophy of pain control contributed significantly to the relative measure of well-being reported by hospice patients. Effects of proper pain control are a high priority item for subsequent research.

Accent on quantity of services can lead to neglect in the measurement of quality of those services. Data collection methods should be designed not only to prove that many activities take place, but also to prove that those activities that took place were or were not effective (7). Program objectives must be based on proved effectiveness and not on unfounded assumptions. Levels of objectives, immediate and ultimate, should not be confused.

Design and utilization of a data retrieval system specifically tailored to meet needs of evaluation of structure and process is a necessity. An evaluation that relies heavily on existing records not only disregards the benefits of research in collection and analysis of data, but also involves the investigator in statistics that are biased or of questionable reliability. Inclusion of a control or comparison group facilitates detection of observable changes due to the program. Without a control group, there is no way of knowing whether changing indices represent program effects and whether those effects are beneficial relative to effects of alternative treatment. Selection of individual activities and the weight those activities are assigned in determining program effects should be based on objective, verifiable criteria. Outcome measures should have proven validity and reliability. The generalizability of results of an evaluation study from a single service facility for others like it depends on comparability of home care program objectives and settings as well as characteristics of the respective communities served (8).

A few empirical studies of specific parameters are currently underway. Dr. Robert Twycross at St. Christopher's in London and Dr. Ronald Melzak at the Royal Victoria Hospital in Montreal are conducting research studies on pain and the use of narcotic mixtures. Dr. Colin Murray Parkes is studying psychosocial effects of hospice care on the bereaved and is developing a protocol for evaluation of the St. Christopher's home care program. Dr. John Hinton is looking at levels of anxiety and depression in St. Christopher's patients as compared with a nonhospice group. However, these are all research studies focusing on one or two parameters of terminal care or bereavement. Aside from measurements used in the evaluation of the hospice in New Haven, there have been no overall systematic evaluation procedures carried out on any hospice program.

One of the reasons for this lack of measurement lies in the history of the hospice movement. The movement arose as a reaction to the poor treatment terminal patients have received in acute care hospitals. Terminal patients have been known to be abused under the auspices of predominantly research-oriented oncology departments. Reaction to such abuse accounts for failure of attempts to introduce true systematic evaluation into British hospices. In New Haven, the director of the evaluation department has spent much time teaching clinical staff the value and importance to the patient and family of producing relevant information. The result has been a close working relationship between the two departments, who cooperate in the gathering of accurate data, and the development of noninvasive instruments for measurement of program effectiveness. Lack of such collaboration and the paucity of program information from Britain have in the past hindered the development of new programs.

Effectiveness of descriptive accounts and case histories in communicating the hospice concept is as indisputable as need for relevant empirical statistical data and measures of program effectiveness in facilitating creation of new programs. Although rigorous, scientifically controlled studies are the ideal, alternative methods must be sought in cases where such studies are not feasible. Preexperimental designs for evaluative research may be resorted to in the event that true experimental studies cannot be executed.

The Buckingham study of the surgical and palliative care wards of the Royal Victoria Hospital is an example of the use of preexperimental methodology (9). Participant observation, the most primitive of preexperimental techniques, was used in examination of patterns of interaction and other complex phenomena of the wards. Findings of the study illustrate the utility of methods used for the detection of complex relationships with no previous research basis. Terminal patients comprised a powerful support system for one another through the sharing and provision of help. Care provided by family members was considered to be extremely important. Student nurses invested much time, care, and interest in terminal patients, thus helping them maintain their selfhood. Patients were perceived as having a need to give and thus maintained their pride in themselves and, consequently, their individuality.

Thus, specific needs of patients and particular shortcomings in the nature of hospital care were detected. However, despite its usefulness as an exploratory technique, participant observation is an inadequate method of program evaluation when more sophisticated alternatives are feasible. However, it is difficult to isolate and develop specific and objective parameters and measurable criteria for evaluation of health services, particularly in the field of terminal care. It is vital that progress that has been made in this area at the hospice in New Haven be adapted and developed in evaluation of other hospice programs.

Evaluation can be viewed as an independent check on the adequacy of hospice program planning. On the other hand, evaluation contributes to the planning phase of program development by delineating problems, resources, and objectives, and by determining rational courses of action. True evaluation research allows determination of the extent to which stated program objectives are met through program activities. Program activities must therefore be reliably recorded, and ultimately, the degree to which results can be attributed to hospice program activities must be determined. Accumulation of specific knowledge regarding needs of the terminally ill is of paramount importance for fostering the work of those charged with patient care. It is in such a manner that findings of evaluative studies will contribute to the well-being of the dying.

References

1. Donabedian, A. Evaluating the quality of medical care. *Milbank Memorial Fund Quarterly*, 1966, *44*(3), 166–203.
2. Buckingham, R. W. Evaluation of the hospice home care program (unpublished doctoral dissertation), 1977.
3. Derogatis, *SCL-90 R Administration, Scoring and Procedures Manual—1.* Clinical Psychometrics Research Unit, Johns Hopkins University School of Medicine, 1977.
4. Weissman, M. M., & Bothwell, S. Assessment of social adjustment by patient self-report. *Archives of General Psychiatry*, 1976, *33*, 1114–1115.
5. Lubin, B. Adjective Checklists for Measurement of Depression. *Archives of General Psychiatry*, 1975, *12*, 57–62.
6. Campbell & Stanley, *Experimental and quasi-experimental designs for research.* Chicago: Rand McNally, 1963.
7. Suchman, E. A. *Evaluative research: Principles and practices in public service and action programs.* New York: Russell Sage Foundation, 1950.
8. Weiss, C. H. *Evaluating action programs: Readings in social action and education.* Boston: Allyn and Bacon, 1972.
9. Buckingham, R. W., Lack, S., Mount, B., MacLean, L., & Collins, J. Living with the dying: Use of the technique of participant observation. *Canadian Medical Association Journal*, 1976, *115*, 1211–1215.

Bibliography

Alkin, M. C. Evaluation theory development. *Evaluation Comment*, 1969, *2*(1), 2–7.
Bateman, W. Assessing program effectiveness: A rating system for identifying relative program success. *Welfare in Review*, 1968, *6*(1), 1–10.
Buckingham, R. W. *A continuing care—at home program for patients with terminal cancer and their families.* Unpublished National Cancer Institute Final Hospice, Inc. Report, October 1977.

Elinson, J. Effectiveness of social action programs in health and welfare. In *Assessing the Effectiveness of Child Health Services, Report of the Fifty-Sixth Russ Conference on Pediatric Research*, 1977, pp. 79–88.

Hagen, E. D., & Thorndike, R. L. Evaluation. In *Encyclopedia of educational research* (3rd ed.). New York: MacMillan, 1960, pp. 482–486.

Herzog, E. *Some guidelines for evaluative research.* Washington, D.C.: Government Printing Office, 1959.

Hyman, H. H., & Wright, C. R. Evaluating social action programs. In P. Lazarsfeld, W. H. Sewell, & H. Wilensky (Eds.), *The uses of sociology*, New York: Basic, 741–782.

Kelman, H. R., & Elinson, J. Strategy and tactics of evaluating a large scale medical program. *Proceedings of the U.S. social statistics section*, Washington, D.C.: American Statistical Association, 1968, 169–191.

Klinegerg, O. The problem of evaluation research. *International Social Science Bulletin*, 1955, 7(3), 347–351.

Schulberg, H. C., & Bater, F. Program evaluation models and the implementation of research findings. *American Journal of Public Health*, 1968, *58*(2), 1248–1255.

Schulberg, H. C., Shadan, A. & Baher, F. *Program evaluation in the health fields.* New York: Behavioral Publications, 1970.

Suchman, E. A. *Evaluative research: Principles and practices in public service and action programs.* New York: Russell Sage Foundation, 1967.

Weiss, C. H. *Evaluating action programs: Readings in social action and education.* Boston: Allyn and Bacon, 1972.

Wilder, D. E. Problems of evaluative research. In *Social Deviance*, London: Tavistock, 1964, 243–273.

Request reprints from Professor Robert W. Buckingham III, Teachers College, Box 114, Columbia University, New York, N.Y. 10027.

∞∞

ISSUES IN CARING

∞∞

∞∞

IN SEARCH OF MODELS OF CARE

∞∞

GLEN W. DAVIDSON
Southern Illinois University, Springfield

*Most hospice programs list "spiritual support" among the charac-
teristics of hospice care, but then avoid defining it except in
ambiguous ways. The author argues that without careful definition
of "spiritual," hospice care will be little different in quality from
that offered in acute and chronic care centers. The "spiritual
quest" is defined as a unifying and integrating process that permits
a human being to be oriented to wholeness or dignity. Also
discussed is the challenge to hospice care staff to defy trends in
recent health care that allow staff rather than patients to determine what dignity means, thereby making the patient an object
rather than a subject.*

The hospice seeks to provide care for the terminally ill and is an
alternative model to other health care institutions whose prior-
ities are either with solely curing diseases (as in hospitals) or
imposing custodial care (as in nursing homes)—both an affront
to human dignity.

A hospice, either as a place or as a service program offered
in a variety of contexts, allows terminally ill patients to
maintain their dignity by controlling pain, offering specialized
nursing care appropriate for the ill person, and providing psychosocial support for the patient and the family as, together, they
adapt to the implications of an ending life. These are seen as the
characteristics of "care" most needed by the terminally ill and
most often abused in other health care institutions.

Despite their common root, the words *hospice* and *hospital*—
meaning hospitality, or extending dignity to guests—are now
seen as distinctions: hospice provides care for the terminally ill

because hospitals are focused on curing the disease of the temporarily ill.

At St. Christopher's Hospice in London, and at most of the hospices in North America, a characteristic of care vaguely identified is "spiritual support." At best, spiritual support is described as respecting the terminally ill person's religious point of view—a stance that has evolved from denominational ecumenism that seems equivalent to political toleration. Spiritual support is also described as that service provided by a chaplain or other person in a religious role—a stance that seems to be ethereal because no one defines what that role does. Or again, spiritual support is presumed to be a quality of care because the institutions where services are provided, or because the staff providing the services, are under religious authority. At worst, spiritual support is ignored because it is presumed to be "strictly personal," "unscientific," or "incapable of being evaluated."

Spiritual refers both to the substance, breath or air, and the activating and essential principle that is life. A classic definition of death is the absence of spirit where material substances are separated from spiritual forces. Spiritual dimensions are the unifying principles of people's lives and while very personal, are also inherently social—"the need to be with others." One may act, according to this definition, with self-awareness or self-consciousness.

If spiritual refers to the unifying and integrating dimensions of living, then spiritual support must refer to those skills that assist patients, families, and staff with their individual and collective efforts to be whole. A staff member's spiritual role is as capable of being evaluated as any other role on the basis of results and the skills for effecting results. With this definition it is possible to examine whether a model of service is also a model of care. It is possible that the model, whether medical, psychological, nursing, or even religious, does not respect the patient's dignity because it tends to alienate rather than unify, confuse rather than integrate life for the sufferer.

Much that has been published on thanatology since 1960 carries the assumption that it is North American culture that is alienating and disorienting. It is argued that the subject of death for most people today is taboo and that contemporary North American culture is death-denying, as though the second assertion follows necessarily from the first. It is also argued that terminally ill patients and their families should accept the inevitable separation and face death as a fact of life. It is as though the vision of what should be—a religious stance—comes from that stereotype of old age when people are tired, accepting, and "ready to go," satisfied that they have lived as best as they can. The fact is that premature dying is the crisis for most terminally ill patients who have yet to finish their struggles of unifying and integrating their responsibilities and desires into a complete and whole life.

I suggest that denial is an appropriate and, for some patients, final characteristic of dignity insofar as it is part of one's spiritual quest. What determines whether the hospice model can provide unique institutional care depends on whether it is the patient rather than staff who defines what care is. In order to understand denial as an inherent part of dignity, it is initially necessary to disassociate it from the assertion that death is a taboo subject.

The subject of death has never been universally taboo in North American culture. By just looking at bibliographies, a person will discover that there has been no dearth of writing on the subject either in the popular or academic presses. What one can see in the literature, however, is how specific assumptions about life and death, and the functions of those assumptions, go unquestioned for a generation or more.

For that generation, specific assumptions are protected from questioning. Questioning specific assumptions about life and death that are held sacred is taboo for those people holding the assumption at the time.

Taboos are presuppositional in character, and are treated as though "sacred and beyond doubt" (1). A taboo is affirmed without question. It is not denied. The misunderstanding, or misuse, of the term has led not only to misunderstanding of the ways death is faced by both patient and practitioner, but also to misdiagnosis of the patient's use of denial.

The propensity to generalize from parochial data that reflect only one discipline or one culture at a specific time in history has already been documented in studies of the "helping professions." Insistence that patients should, rather than may, be "pain free," "be happy," "be reunited with all of their relatives," or "die accepting their fate" can, separated from an individual patient's spiritual context, be as parochial and may be used as defense mechanisms imposed by hospice staff to protect their taboos about dying.

If some models for care of the ill have based conclusions on unexamined hypotheses, so too have they consistently ignored the structures in society and culture that organize both the functions and meanings of life at a presuppositional level. Some structures of meaning are held to be sacred by many members of a society or culture and are beyond doubt; they are hallowed tradition, and therefore not open to question and examination (2).

Presuppositions drawn from society and culture are inherent in anyone's spiritual quest because they are what we trust. The health care worker can beyond doubt trust methods of science, view humans as having both conscious and unconscious characters, and affirm "death" as a part of reality, while meeting questioning any one of these with scorn, ridicule, or lack of acknowledgment. But to do so is only to reveal what is affirmed, what is taboo, not what is denied.

Our presuppositions are taboo for us because we have trusted their truth and committed our energies and interests as though free to get on with the discovery, examination, and rediscovery of their implications. Even though our presuppositions can be questioned by others, for us to question their truth is taboo. To summarize, a taboo is affirmed without question. While the subject of death itself is not taboo, specific assumptions about death are held to be beyond questioning by people at a given time in history.

Denial, that is, the refusal to admit the truth of something or the declaration that something is not so, does not necessarily follow the affirmation of a taboo. It follows the challenge to a taboo, the examination of and interpretation about its sacredness, and the calling of its truth into question. In the diagnosis of denial, our methods of interpretation must make a primary distinction between a subject that itself is taboo, and the manner of addressing a sacred subject that is considered the "only appropriate way." A secondary distinction must be made between behavior that refuses to face a taboo because of the subject's awesomeness, and behavior that is the result of having been repulsed by the manner in which the object's sacredness is addressed.

Of what importance are these distinctions? Their importance is based on what seems to be the commonly accepted goal of care for the terminally ill, namely that a patient has the right to die with dignity. *Dignity* means that a person, even though in the process of dying, is addressed as having status of worth and is treated in ways of honor. Patients are the subject of dignity. Health care staffs are responders to the subjects. It is the patient's taboos that must be respected if the patient is to have dignity. This distinction is forced by the rediscoveries that pluralistic societies exist in North America. It does not take extensive analysis of interviews with the terminally ill to realize that patient populations in large, modern-day hospitals, nursing homes, or hospice programs represent the cultural pluralism of North American society. Unlike past ages when patients could defend their own sense of dignity because they were treated at home, today's patients report that the hospitals and nursing homes are foreign territory where they seldom feel at home or have a sense of dignity. Unification and integration of life's experiences are difficult there. The mores, rhythms, and values used by professional health care workers to do their work tend to be imposed on the patient. Will the same occur in a hospice?

Interviews with terminally ill patients have revealed that the patient uses denial inconsistently. For example, to a person such as the physician or the spouse, the patient will avoid the subject of the terminal illness. Yet to another person such as a sympathetic friend, nurse, psychiatrist, or chaplain, the patient will be quite open. It is as though it is not appropriate to share some realizations with certain people that are shared with others. One reason is that all too often patients' sense of propriety has been violated by those with whom they "deny." Patients deny when their taboos are transgressed or they have been repulsed by the way others have addressed their taboos while trying to protect their own. It can be said of us all that "there are moments when he suddenly realizes that he is no longer reacting emotionally to events, experiences, and activities that would once have terrified, shamed, or upset him deeply (3, pp. 30–34). Clinicians tend to forget patients' perceptions of propriety because they have forgotten their own as their professional roles developed. The ways practitioners act out roles, the manner with which terminal illness is treated by relatives of the patient, and the context that an institution provides may be perceived by patients as alienating and disorienting. From patients' perspectives, their spiritual quest is thwarted.

Examination of interviews with the terminally ill frequently reveal that physicians, psychiatrists, nurses, ministers, or social workers, even though they see themselves as sympathetic, tend to impose their own presuppositions of propriety on the dying patient—dignity as defined and generalized by the methods of the respective disciplines. As Neale (4) tactfully put it, "we are prone to have powerful and rigid opinions on matters relating to death. We are prone to enforce these opinions on others." In an age when the ethics of care for terminally ill patients are in question, in roles where human feelings have been suppressed by professional demeanor, in surroundings more familiar to practitioners than patients, dignity tends to be defined by and for the health care worker rather than the patient. It is the health care worker's taboos and methodological presuppositions that are honored. And a patient's denial is behavior that refuses to acknowledge the practitioner's taboos rather than behavior that refuses to account for, or cannot accept, a certain reality about the patient. The following case history (5) illustrates my point.

A Gypsy male was admitted to university hospital with advanced cancer of the lungs. He was approximately 45 years of age, father of five children, and variously employed. Despite the fact that a large number of Gypsies soon gathered in the hospital lobby to express concern about him, thereby making the patient's presence an irregular occurrence in the hospital's routine, the case history recorded at the time read:

Pureto Rican male shows contempt for his condition, persists in smoking, and frequently violates care plan. Roman Catholic. On welfare. Easily excited and very nervous. Recommend no visitors.

The patient's nervousness had become acute and he refused to cooperate with the care plan for him. Despite the nurse's efforts to prevent him from having tobacco, he somehow managed several puffs a day before the cigarette could be taken away from him. He had, according to his medical history, started smoking at around the age of 3 months. He would die smoking. The attending physician requested a psychiatric consultation for the patient. The psychiatrist reported:

Patient exhibits extensive denial. Practicing Roman Catholic who seems obsessed with his own immortality. Talks about going on a journey to get away from it all. Seems confused as to place and time of trip. Presence of visitors seems to accentuate condition.

Visitors had been restricted, but because of the large hospital population, a few Gypsies always managed to get into the patient's room undetected. Even small children managed a visit. As the health care staff increasingly found themselves in an adversary position, the Gypsies became antagonized and destructive. Finally, they were confronted by the head of hospital security. One of the Gypsies assumed the role of spokesman. He announced that the patient was "Son of the Gypsy King" and the visitors were his followers who had a right to be with him.

In contrast to the aloof, ready to stereotype, disdainful attitudes expressed toward him by the health care staff, the patient was now stereotyped as "the Gypsy prince." Nurses fluttered in and out of his room. Doctors came to examine and reexamine him. Even the hospital administrator managed to see what the "distinguished visitor" needed, and ordered that one whole waiting room be reserved for the Gypsies on the ground floor. That helped with security anyway, because the whole group could be watched by closed circuit TV. The patient had been treated as a hostile intruder by the health care staff previously. Now he was receiving top care of the house.

The stereotype, with its own perspective of dignity, functioned in a new way. Members of the staff began reporting that hospital equipment disappeared and that the reserved waiting room looked like a "pig's sty." After the Gypsies departed, the head of security confessed that the missing equipment had mysteriously reappeared or was found to be in the hospital's repair shops where the equipment had been sent several weeks before the patient's arrival. He could think of nothing reported missing which could be attributed to the Gypsies' fingers. But the stereotype functioned both for the benefit of the patient, who received better care, and for the Gypsies as a whole, who used the staff's predisposed assumptions about them to advantage. No *gadje*—non-Gypsy—came into the "sty," and that meant the Gypsies could feel more at home. The gadje's attitude turned from one of disdain to one of fear which meant that only "authorities" communicated with them. That gave the Gypsies a sense of importance, negative as it was, which is always better in such situations than to be ignored. Despite all of the privileged treatment given the patient, however, all visitors except the group's spokesman were still restricted from entering his room. And the patient continued to be uncooperative and aggressive.

A multidisciplinary team was organized to reinterview the patient. They began the interview by asking the patient which of his needs were not being met in the hospital. He replied that he wanted more tobacco because he wasn't "so nervous" when he smoked.

Q: "What is it that makes you nervous?"
R: "Everything about this here place."

Q: "Can you think of anything else that might calm you?"
R: "I need my people here."

Q: "You need your people here in your room to help you be calm?"
R: "Yes."

Q: "The nurses have told us that you seem more nervous when you have visitors. Is that correct?"
R: "I'm nervous when gadje are here. And I'm nervous when my people are kicked out. We can't be natural together."

For a Gypsy, whose identity is so deeply established as a member of a corporate people, to be separated from them at any time of crisis is a threat to security. Hospital procedure required that only two visitors be permitted in any patient's room at one time and in the case of this patient, no visitors were officially permitted. Upon recommendation of the interviewing team, the patient was moved next to the waiting room where the Gypsies could circulate in and out of his room.

The psychiatrist had characterized the patient's behavior as "extensive denial." The patient was resistive in the interview. He refused to follow the care plan prescribed. He spoke of going on a trip when it was obvious he would not walk out of the hospital. What else but *ego-immortalis?* It was all in Freud's works!

The psychiatric analysis was wrong and the care plan was arbitrary. For the next few days, the Gypsies circulated in and out, encouraging the patient to ready for his trip. What became obvious was that the trip was a euphemism for death. As the psychiatrist had done, the Gypsies were using metaphors to speak of anticipated events in future time yet to be experienced. In classical cultural form, the Gypsies spoke of a journey across the river that encircles the world as they conceive it—a view similar to the myth of Choron and the river Styx. What the psychiatrist had taken in the first interview as a sign of denial was the patient's symbolic reference to his destiny, for which appropriate preparation was vital. The hospital's procedures and the staff's ignorance of the patient's cultural contexts of reference thwarted the patient from appropriately dealing with the reality of his situation.

Death was symbolized by the river, the crossing of which requires preparation. For the Gypsy patient, preparation required saying goodbye to all the relatives, settling of disputes, entrusting his wife and children to other's care, and dividing responsibilities among the strong. As each of these concerns was cared for, the language of denial was used less and less. When hospital procedures thwarted this process, the patient and the other Gypsies tended toward panic. They feared that they would not be able to accomplish what is, for them, vital if one is to die correctly. Their sense of dignity required rituals they deemed necessary to complete one's destiny. Denial, in multiple forms, was the ritualized attempts to hold off time long enough to complete the patient's business with his people.

The Gypsies know themselves as "man" among "strangers." Much that exemplifies evil comes to them through "strangers." To have surrounded the patient at the end with gadje, busy taking pulse or performing heroic measures for sustaining vital signs, would have prevented the patient from being with his people. It would have been understood by him as "hell"— alienation from those who affirm his sense of dignity. A sensitive report on his medical chart read: "The patient needs to die among his own kind."

The case history of the Gypsy patient is told here to illustrate how we can misidentify denial when we do not understand patients' spiritual frames of reference. It is a warning for us to approach patients' metaphors with respect and caution. No more than the scientist does the nonprofessional use metaphor for projecting imagination into future time. No less than the scientist does the nonprofessional use metaphors rooted on past experience to articulate expectations for the future. Scientists as professionals use a careful codification of metaphor and symbol to communicate with their peers. But scientists as human beings resort to the language of metaphor and symbol from traditions of culture to communicate with loved ones. How else do they speak affectionately to others and have communicated to them a sense of dignity?

The case history may be insightful for understanding why metaphors of denial are used by patients with some people, but not with others even in a relatively short span of time. When health care personnel are perceived as strangers, they are, in the mind of patients, part of that against which they are struggling to maintain a sense of dignity. To thwart patients by violating frames of reference may cause the staff to become a symbol of evil, of frustration, or even, ultimately, of chaos. What more is there for humans to fight than chaos when they confront death?

The metaphors and symbols patients use for order and chaos, good and evil, right and wrong, and fulfillment and frustration come from their personal and cultural experiences. Sigmund Freud appreciated, analyzed, and used metaphors and symbols. He (6) explored the use of the symbol, "immortality," and linked it as an explanation for the horrors of World War I. Warriors can commit their acts of barbarism, he thought, because they do not believe they, themselves, will be killed. Their acts, he continued, intrude into "our conventional attitude toward death." For barbarian and civilian alike, the conventional attitude to which he referred was, that while everyone acknowledges owing "a debt to Nature and must expect to pay the reckoning," in reality we display "an unmistakable tendency to 'shelve' death, to eliminate it from life" (p. 761). Here, Freud spoke with historical sensitivity.

One of the pressing questions of intellectuals in late 18th century European society was whether people had something immortal about their natures. Is there something of abiding value that characterizes an individual, yet transcends death? Parlor society then prominent in Europe assumed that there is. The new science, logical positivism, and the war raised serious doubts. Yet, for most learned people, the whole drive toward "being civilized" continued to be based upon the assumption that some value permeated the order of the universe.

Freud saw in his people's aspirations for transcendence, and their attempts to find within themselves something of permanent worth, evidence of both humanity's conscious denial of mortality and unconscious inability to grasp personal finitude. He deduced that this was the case because no one personally could have previously experienced death. And he spoke of inexperience of death as synonymous with immortality. I want to suggest that humanity has no experience of immortality either. But everyone has frequent experiences of changing in such ways that it is internalized into their own identities as dying. And most people, even those of whom Freud wrote, distinguish between their own death at the end of maturity and the possibilities of their own premature death. What Freud was doing, it seems to me, was taking the symbol common to his own people in his own time and presupposing that it was universal. His "thoughts for the times" were made into "thoughts for *all* time!"

Individual immortality was the focus of near obsession, particularly in late 18th century European arts, religion, and literature. But the obsession was fading by the time of Freud's adult life. He also ignored the studies of cultures even then available to him which showed the parochial usage of the symbol in Europe. Not only is the concept of individual immortality not universal, there are but few cultures in the world that maintain a myth of individual immortality.

Freud used the symbol of *immortality* as a synonym for one's end. But a distinction needs to be made. *End,* when understood in the sense of the Greek word, *telos,* refers to purpose of destiny or fulfillment of design. Insofar as individual behavior is rooted in the identity of a people, individuals assess meaning by how well they have met the requirements of their people's destiny; for example, has an individual reached that development of life expected of the mature person? End, when understood in the sense of the Latin word, *finis,* refers to termination or cessation. It is not a contradiction for a person to seek a telos and yet accept personal finis. And the presence of both ends seems to be more consistent with the descriptive data ascribed to the unconscious than the conclusions Freud reached. The failure to make such a distinction leads us to see humanity's quest for destiny solely as denial of mortality, when denial of mortality may be used for a purpose other than to assert one's immortality. How, then, can we discover the ways a patient uses denial in the face of death, and how is dignity to be defined? The answers must come from each patient. Those interviews for me that have been most fruitful for discovering these answers have been conducted by a multidisciplinary team—with a psychiatrist, social worker, psychiatric nurse, or chaplain. I am repeatedly impressed with the unexpected and more open responses that are stimulated. Also a colleague trained in a specialty different from mine, balances my tendencies to look only for the data most interesting to me. The implications can be decisive.

I interview on the assumption that people receive from their culture the stories of identity that give them the symbols by which they explain where they came from (myth of origin),[1]

---

[1] I use *myth* as a technical word that refers to the stories a people tell about themselves to explain who they are. Myths, contrary to popular usage, are not

where they are going (myth of destiny), and how they are to get there (myth of vocation). Individuals discover the boundaries of their separate identities through participation in the cultural rituals of their people that reveal paradigmatic models for thought and action. For example, I take it that the people about whom Freud wrote as being shocked by the behavior of the warriors had so come to accept their "civilized ways" of thinking about death that this behavior was deeply offensive even though based on the same symbol. I understand ritual to mean habits of thought and action that become symbolic and relate persons to their people's myths of origin and destiny. Rituals not only reveal but permit access to that "right order" that creates and fulfills life (telos). Consequently, "the ways we handle this" often become inviolable for both patient and practitioner. To question "the way" is taboo.

Having now personally participated in, observed, or reviewed the tape recordings of over 1,200 interviews with adults who were terminally ill, I have come to several conclusions. First, even though patients were frequently unaware of where they learned what they considered "appropriate behavior," almost all of the interviewed patients acted out rituals that used myths and symbols identifiable with a culture. It is as though once a pattern of action is sacralized, no thought is given to its purpose or origin as long as its efficacy is not rejected. It is presuppositional. Second, no matter how estranged terminally ill patients were with staff, family, friends, or society, they acted ritually in an effort to maintain or to recover a sense of order. This is the spiritual quest. Third, depending on how patients assessed their own situations, they chose a specific kind of ritual from among competing and contradictory possibilities to meet their specific needs. Fourth, there is often contradictory assessment about the meaning of dignity between those who are actually dying and those who are still healthy but are in the presence of the terminally ill.

Carl Nighswonger (7) has given the helpful term *drama* to the ritualized behavior of the terminally ill. It is an appropriate

understood as illusions or as fantasies by the people using them but as sacred truths. The telling of myth is to speak of a taboo in an appropriate way.

term, I believe, because it conveys the patients' awareness that they are in a struggle, between an order around which their lives have been organized, and possibilities of chaos in the unknown future. For many of the patients, their situation was seen as a battle between what they held as meaningful in life and what they feared would destroy their hope of destiny. Each drama is a battle for resolution between what for them is good and evil. Resolution comes when patients find an appropriate paradigm for handling the situation and the questions it generates. It is as though patients were saying that they could, covertly or overtly, establish themselves in a paradigmatic state to which they and their people are destined, if patients are able to maintain access to the roots of their identities. It is the seeming attempt to reproduce, in the microcosm of patients' situations, the system of rhythmic and reciprocally conditioning influences that characterizes and constitutes "right order," even when their notion of "right order" was in conflict with that of physicians, nurses, social workers, clergy, or family.

A "drama of shock" is acted out when routine, or what the individual calls "normal life," is threatened by radical disruption. The threat of impending death is the most radical disruption of all if the individual is not ready to die. When an individual or society is shocked, the occasion is met by rituals either of denial or panic. *Denial* is what has been called the human shock absorber to tragedy. It is a way in which emotions are desensitized sufficiently to permit suspending the sense of time and, thereby to delay the approach of death. This permits the individual to "have time" to marshall resources and to search for the appropriate response, to search for the right paradigm in the face of overwhelming chaos, and to seek to recover wholeness.

Panic is acting out the fear that the disruption has made life chaotic. The structures of stability and the routine rituals of living that have permitted a sense of order now seem unreal. Panic may take the form of hysteria, psychosis, or suicide, but whatever the form, to the person in panic the real world has come apart.

Inherent to the drama of shock is the fear of losing something vital for destiny or telos. What one fears may be lost appears to be heavily influenced by cultural presuppositions.

This is seen clearly when the symbol, or symbols, of "right order" are threatened. The symbol is different among peoples and, to a lesser degree, different among members of a people. Many persons, for example, have made "right order" and "peaceful dying" synonymous, and the possibility raised by radical disruption, e.g., that they will die in terror, to them, is to have to die in "hell." And they will mislead relatives and health care staff about their awareness of their condition if that is what is necessary in order to die in peace. Yet, for others, to die pain free or peaceful is out of order.

Whatever the presuppositions of "right order," denial as a behavioral pattern is used as a ritual to suspend time until the ways appropriate for handling the crisis can be determined. When those ways can be followed and respected by the health care staff and relatives, the patient dies with dignity. Rather than being the consequence of a disabusing process, dignity comes from the sense of what patients acknowledge as appropriate for their end (finis) within the context of their people's destiny (telos). If patients are to be honored as individuals, they deserve no less and can be given nothing better.

Conclusion

The hospice movement seeks to provide care for terminally ill patients that affirms their dignity and is not readily available in health care institutions commited to cure of disease. How ironic that a distinction between *care* and *cure* can be made when both words have a common root! The separation occurred when, what Foucault (8) calls, the "clinical gaze" or perspective developed in 19th century Western thought in conjunction with the historical development of the clinic. Then attention shifted from the person feeling symptoms as the subject to the clinician diagnosing disease and pain as the subject. And the role of curé, healer of souls, became more sharply a competing influence for the patient who has been relegated to the role of object. Yet it was and is the patient's spiritual quest, as subject, which holds care and cure together to mean healing. It was and is respect for the patient's effort to be whole, whatever that means to the patient as a unifying and integrating force of living that defines dignity.

Hospice is a metaphor that attempts to link the needs of the terminally ill patient, the family, and the staff, with that medieval religious institution of hospitality where a community assisted the vulnerable traveler at points of great danger. The hospice movement in North America may be able to provide badly needed and unique care to those faced with terminal illness if that traveler/patient is able to avoid having a shattered identity and is able to recover or maintain a sense of destiny. That is spiritual support.

But what promise is there when one helping role is asserted above another; or the helping roles are presented as subjects; or the patient's efforts at wholeness are reduced to pathological fragments; or service to the needy is romanticized; or death is advertised arrogantly as domesticated?

So long as spiritual support is ill-defined and vague there is little hope that any better care will be provided the vulnerable patient who, as the traveler of old, may be beset by both the viscious and the well-meaning, but thwarted by either from reaching his or her destiny. Health care providers have already demonstrated that facilities, personnel, and other resources can be organized. Whether these can be provided as responses to the patient in quest of uniting and integrating care is at issue.

References

1. Davidson, G. W. Histories and rituals of destiny: Implications for thanatology. *Soundings*, 1971, *54*, 415-434.
2. Parsons, T., & Lidz, W. Death in American society. In E. S. Shneidman (Ed.), *Essays in self-destruction*, New York: Science, 1967.
3. Keniston, K. The medical student. *The New Physician*, 1968, *15*, 30-34. Originally published 1967.
4. Neale, R. E. Psychiatry and religion: Death. *Archives of the Foundation of Thanatology*, 1970, *2*(4), 203.
5. Davidson, G. W. "Gypsies": People with a hidden history. *Soundings*, 1973, *56*, 83-97.
6. Freud, S. *The major works of Sigmund Freud.* Chicago: Encyclopaedia Britannica, 1952.

7. Nighswonger, C. A. Ministry to the dying as a learning encounter. *Journal of Thanatology*, 1971, *1*(2), 101–108.

8. Foucault, M. [The birth of the clinic: An archaeology of medical perception.] (A. M. Sheridan Smith, trans.), New York: Pantheon, 1973. Originally published 1963.

Request reprints from Glen W. Davidson, Ph.D., Southern Illinois University School of Medicine, P.O. Box 3926, Springfield, Ill. 62708.

THE ETHICS OF TERMINAL CARE

GEORGE J. AGICH

Southern Illinois University, Springfield

The need for a critical and analytical approach to the ethics of terminal care is suggested by considering a series of unexamined questions regarding the justification of terminal care. Among them are: (1) Do patients have a right to terminal care? (2) What qualifies personnel to provide terminal care? (3) Do we really know what "care," a "good death," or "accepting one's death" mean? (4) Are assumptions about the hospice model contradictory to the demands of scientific research? If terminal care is, as many seem to believe, a moral and ethical enterprise, then such considerations must be given a more prominent place in discussions of the hospice movement.

The term *ethics* has three different but related usages: (1) a *pattern* of life or conduct, (2) a *set of rules* of conduct, and (3) an *inquiry* about patterns of life and rules of conduct. It is with this latter characterization of ethics as inquiry that we are concerned.

So characterized, ethics is preeminently a critical and reflective enterprise that is philosophical in nature. It is concerned with reasons and arguments that justify courses of action, rather than with the style or pattern of action or with a set of rules of conduct per se. In this regard, the phrase *ethics of terminal care* signifies an inquiry into the style of care provided for the terminally ill and the arguments justifying that care as well as the codes and moral principles, explicit or implicit, that shape the style of care.

Discussions of terminal care often include what can be generously read as ethical or value dimensions, even though these discussions seldom develop a sustained, much less systematic, inquiry into value presuppositions. In what may be globally characterized as the hospice movement, certain facts are presented in a way that make it appear that hospice care is ethically justified as a response to a series of problems facing medicine.

For instance, it is often noted that acute care facilities tend to be characterized by impersonality—by a technical rather than a human approach to patients. The style of delivering care in such facilities contributes both to anonymity of staff members as well as to isolation of patients from health care providers. In short, acute care facilities are structured to effectively care for acute medical and surgical problems, but not the needs of dying patients. The style of care in these settings is therefore seen as basically insensitive to the special needs of the dying patient (1, 2). So, without directly analyzing and criticizing the style of acute care, an alternative model—hospice care—is proposed for terminally ill patients.

This model includes a protocol for pain alleviation different from that common in medical practice (3-5), an active role for the family in caring for the dying patient (6), as well as an open and nontechnically oriented staff and institutional operation (7). But while there is a clear difference in style and a commitment to different rules of conduct, this difference is not self-justificatory of hospice care. In fact, the most significant mistake in the literature on terminal care is the belief that this difference of style comprises the main ethical issue in terminal care—shift the patient from one environment to another and the main ethical problems of terminal care are settled. This solution is easy only because it is simpleminded.

After all, even if one agrees that modern scientific medicine has failed the terminally ill, one might rationally conclude either that nothing ought to be done for these patients even though the situation is lamentable or that what must be done will take a different course than the strategies that mark the hospice movement. Without arguing either of these two alternatives, it should be clear that further premises are necessary to make the move from description and evaluation of the circumstances of acute care and hospice care to justification for a specific course of action. However, these premises have been largely presupposed in the literature on terminal care, particularly in the discussions of administrative and institutional aspects of that care (8).

In part because the hospice movement is concerned with institutional changes in order to alter delivery of medical services to terminally ill patients, two sets of contrasting ideas seem to differentiate styles of care encouraged by the hospice movement and by acute medical and surgical units: cure versus care and normality versus well-being. This contrast is significant and complex.

Modern medical institutions are designed for the purpose of curing disease. Patients are cast in the sick role and sick behavior is reinforced by hospital procedures (9). The patient is expected to want to get well and to cooperate freely with health care personnel pursuant to that end. In effect, the system is geared to diagnosing and curing patients of specific disease states in order to return the patient to a state of normal functioning. Normal functioning is defined in terms of social expectations via the sick role and in terms of medical and biological considerations of function and structure. Because these expectations are fairly clear, patients have a definite role structured for them. Whatever inconveniences exist in the hospital space, for instance a regimented life style, diagnostic testing, and the pain and nuisance of treatment modalities, they are tolerated because they are seen as contributory to generally accepted ends of cure and normality.

In contrast to these regulative ideas, the hospice offers the ideas of care and well-being. Care is directed toward a patient. It is not a technical skill, procedure, or drug that is intended to eradicate a specifically diagnosed abnormality; rather, care is the quality of ministering to a sick individual. The purpose of such ministering is not to restore the individual to some scientifically predetermined and socially accepted state of normality, but to help the individual recover a state of well-being. To be sure, cure and care are not properly separate in medical practice, yet they can be fruitfully distinguished for the sake of argument and are so distinguished in the literature on terminal care. However, there are problems with this distinction that can be made clear by considering the term *health,* which ambiguously bridges the notions of normality and well-being.

Health is commonly used to mean both normality and well-being. The difference in these two usages relates not only to the context of care, but to the meaning of that care (10). For instance, health understood as normality relates to general psychological and biological norms of functioning that are applied to individuals. The disease—the specific abnormality that a patient has—is treated for the purpose of cure. In this framework care (another ambiguous term) tends to be reduced to cure. Health as well-being, on the other hand, refers to other norms. Physical normality may be a constitutent of health as well-being, but well-being cannot be reduced to it. For, what is good for an individual or proper to an individual includes more than physical normality. Hence, care allows a wider scope of action than cure insofar as it includes ideals other than the norms of biological and psychological functioning. And here precisely is the problem: The legitimate limits on action are not as clear in the case of hospice care as in the context of medical cure, because the ideals of well-being are largely undefined. For this reason difficulties emerge.

Hospice care is ostensibly defined from the patient's perspective, in terms of the patient's need rather than the system of medical knowledge. This shift in perspective carries with it unexamined presuppositions that underscore the necessity of including "the ethics of terminal care" in discussions of hospice care. This need can be illustrated in a series of questions focusing on assumptions of hospice care.

The first problem is perhaps crucial for hospice units—allocation of resources. We have developed the difference between terminal care and acute hospital care in terms of the different ideas guiding patient care: care/well-being and cure/normality. Both sets of ideas are part of the tradition and rhetoric of medicine, though the former set is not part of the reality of medical practice as the hospice movement has shown for at least one class of patients. Given this circumstance, how should hospice care be conceived for the purpose of resource allocation? Is hospice care a medical or health (remember the ambiguity of this notion) need or something different? Thus far, there has been little serious attention to this sort of question. Instead, the concern has been with immediate problems such as third party reimbursement for services (8), but beneath these pragmatic considerations are ethical questions that must be asked:

1. Do patients have a right to terminal care? If there is such a right, what does it mean? For instance, does the alleged right to terminal care imply a moral duty or is it supererogatory, related more to virtues such as compassion and charity than to justice or equity? Another way of expressing this question is to ask whether the right is a moral or social and legal right. Thus far, discussions of terminal care have presupposed that terminal care is part of a right to health or a right to health care as if these notions were themselves unproblematic. However, an ample literature on this subject refutes that preconception (11, pp. 452–465). Relative to the question of the right to health care is the question of the obligation or duty to provide such services. The policy problem of deciding which obligations are to be met when resources are not adequate to meet all needs has hardly been addressed in the literature. Instead, there is the belief that terminal care constitutes a legitimate claim on the health care budget, but little clarification of the grounds of that claim are provided.

2. In addition to the policy aspects of resource allocation, there are personal and personnel problems. For instance, what qualifies personnel to provide terminal care? If the obligation for terminal care is social, then a general or legal answer might be given to the question of the qualifications to provide such care. Skills, required courses of training, etc., could be specified in delineating specific social roles in terminal care. Responsibility for care would then be divided into specific tasks and the allocation of personnel and their accountability could be made on that basis. But what if terminal care is personal as the literature seems to suggest rather than social and task-oriented? Can an institution delegate responsibility in such circumstances in order to assure a quality level of care? In more immediate terms, what role can or should

administrators play in structuring delivery of care and
who is qualified to fill delivery positions? In political
terms, these questions amount to asking who should have
the power to run hospice units and to make policy as
well as day-to-day practical decisions. Should or must
physicians run hospice units rather than nurses, for
instance? It is fair to say that these questions have not
been adequately addresssed by those who enthusiastically
stress the personal commitment aspect of terminal care.
The organization of units, it would seem, has been
determined mainly by economic and political considerations rather than ethical.

A second set of ethical problems relates to the goal or goals
of hospice care. Care and well-being indicate the style but not
the substance of such units. This emphasis is given, in part,
because of the belief that medicine's commitment to
science and technologically-oriented care is inadequate and insensitive to needs of the dying patient. Instead, a different style of
treating dying patients is advocated. But terminal care is not just
style, it involves concrete strategies and tactics for meeting needs
of dying patients. How does one move from considerations of
style to substance, from rhetoric to action?

Needs are never entirely prima facie, but are grounded in
choices, perceptions, and knowledge that relate to our ideals or
goals. In this regard, we are concerned only with the grounds of
knowledge upon which terminal care is based and the issues
involved in developing and enhancing that knowledge base.

For medicine, research is a clear and consistent obligation
insofar as cure and normality imply an idea of action grounded
and validated in scientific knowledge. In this context, we now
understand, at least in a general way, what constitutes legitimate
research and how patients' rights are to be protected. But things
are not so clear in connection with the terminally ill, since in
terminal care emphasis is upon care and well-being. For example,
how are particular services to be justified? In medicine they are
justified by reference to the goal of cure. But in terminal care
the goal is ambiguous since patients' needs are always individual
in nature; so, perhaps, there really is no single model of such

care, but a series of models reflecting different ideals. Thus, do we really know what *care* or a *good death* or what *accepting one's death* mean? Without analysis and argument, do we know that the general use of the Brompton mixture is ethically justified? Discussion of the Brompton mixture has focused on pharmacological aspects and clinical effectiveness, but not the question of the moral status of pain and suffering in dying patients. In terms of what ends or purposes are such practices instituted and how are they justified?

Even if we assume that hospice care will not permit any research unrelated to the dying process, difficult ethical questions still remain. Can the model of care and well-being be adapted without contradiction to the demands of scientific investigation (16–18)? Under this model (or models) patients are treated as persons, that is, as ends in themselves, rather than instrumentally. They are not to be used in any way. Their needs set the goal for care. In this context, then, is research of any sort permissible? The fact that research is regularly conducted within hospice settings on the quality of hospice care, on stages of the dying process, and on the grief and bereavement process does not trivialize this question, but only makes it more pressing. For one can always ask in such cases: Is such study ethically justifiable? That is to say, what rights do terminally ill individuals and their families have that must be protected and recognized in studies of the care of the terminally ill? Or, expressed in more general terms, what is the good or purpose that should be pursued by and for such patients and families?

The notions of care and well-being may surely have the proper feel; however, they require analysis in order to answer our question. It is simply too easy to say that dying patients have the right to easy and painless deaths, a right to have their families actively involved in delivering care, a right to avoid routine diagnostic testing and other.disturbances, and a right to receive emotional support and comfort. But are these basic rights or are they derived from others such as the right to care and well-being? If they are derived, the need to spell out the meaning of care and well-being becomes all the more pressing.

Finally, should patients be "worked through" to the acceptance of death? In part, the question is ethical and conceptual,

but it is also empirical in that an answer must accommodate our
knowledge of the dying process. But how is this knowledge to
be gained? The notion of the "privilege of the sick" must figure
significantly in the question of the ethics of research involving
the dying patient (19, pp. 1–31). The quality of consent must
be subject to suspicion in circumstances where emotional support or attention, even if received solely as an experimental
subject, is highly desired. Finally, can persons or institutions
committed to ideals of care and well-being conduct research
without compromising their basic moral stand? To be sure,
enhancing the knowledge base for terminal care is important,
but does the obligation to expand knowledge in this care
properly belong to the providers of such care?

These questions are of a kind not currently addressed in
discussions of terminal care. In part, this is understandable since
these questions fundamentally ask for a clarification and justification of the idea of the care of the terminally ill, an idea still
in the formative stages. But if terminal care is, as many seem to
believe, a moral and ethical enterprise, then such considerations
must be given a more prominent place. I hope that these general
questions can serve as a guide.

References

1. Netsky, M. Dying in a system of "good care": Case report and
   analysis. *Connecticut Medicine*, 1977, *41*, 33–36.
2. Kohn, J. Hospice movement provides humane alternative for terminally
   ill patients. *Modern Health Care*, 1976, 25–28.
3. Mount, B. M., Ajemian, I., & Scott, J. R. Use of the Brompton
   mixture in treating the chronic pain of malignant disease. *Canadian
   Medical Association Journal*, 1976, *115*, 122–124.
4. Melzack, R., Ofiesh, J. G., & Mount, B. M. The Brompton mixture:
   Effects on pain in cancer patients. *Canadian Medical Association Journal*,
   1976, *115*, 125–129.
5. Schulz, R. Meeting the three major needs of the dying patient.
   Geriatrics, 1976, *31*, 132–137.
6. Craven, J., & Wald, F. Hospice care for dying patients. *American
   Journal of Nursing*, 1975, *75*, 1816–1822.
7. Kohn, J. Hospice building speaks on many emotional levels to patient,
   family. *Modern Health Care*, 1976, *6*, 56–57.
8. Ryder, C. F., & Ross, D. Terminal care issues and alternatives. *Public
   Health Reports*, 1977, *92*, 20–28.

9. Noyes, R., & Clancy, J. The dying role: Its relevance to improved patient care. *Psychiatry,* 1977, *40,* 41–47.
10. Kass, L. R. Regarding the use of medicine and the pursuit of health. *The Public Interest,* 1975, *40,* 11–42.
11. Fried, C. An analysis of "equality" and "rights" in medical care. In R. Hunt & J. Arras (Eds.), *Ethical issues in modern medicine.* Palo Alto: Mayfield, 1977.
12. Sigerist, H. Socialized medicine. *The Yale Review,* 1938, *27,* 481.
13. Szasz, T. S. The right to health. *Georgetown Law Journal,* 1969, *57,* 734–751.
14. Sade, R. M. Medical care as a right: A refutation. *New England Journal of Medicine,* 1971, *285,* 1288–1292.
15. Chapman, C. B., & Talmadge, J. M. The evolution of the right to health concept in the United States. *Pharos,* 1971, *34,* 30–51.
16. Buckingham, R. W., Lack, S. A., Mount, B. M., Maclean, L. D., & Collins, J. T. Living with the dying: Use of the technique of participant observation. *Canadian Medical Association Journal,* 1976, *115,* 1211–1215.
17. Murray, W. B., & Buckingham, R. W. Implications of participant observation in medical studies. *Canadian Medical Association Journal,* 1976, *115,* 1187–1190.
18. Redlich, F. The anthropologist as observer. *The Journal of Nervous and Mental Diseases,* 1973, *157,* 313–319.
19. Jonas, H. Philosophical reflections on experimenting with human subjects. In P. A. Freund (Ed.), *Experimentation with human subjects,* New York: Braziller, 1970.

Request reprints from George J. Agich, Ph.D., Southern Illinois University School of Medicine, P.O. Box 3926, Springfield, Ill. 62708.

∞∞∞

DEATH WITH DIGNITY:
A TRIPARTITE LEGAL RESPONSE

∞∞∞

THEODORE RAYMOND LEBLANG
Southern Illinois University, Springfield

*In attempting to provide a remedy to the legal problems confront-
ing both the terminally ill patient and health care provider, three
legal vehicles have been advanced for consideration and implementation—the living will, the antidysthanasia contract, and right to
die legislation. Of the three, right to die legislation has proven to
be the most effective in permitting the terminally ill patient to
have a significant role in determining the time and manner of
death. This article provides a descriptive overview of the legal
problems that attend medical treatment of the terminally ill
patient as well as a careful analysis of the legal vehicles that have
been offered in response to these problems.*

Introduction

The concept of death with dignity has been given significant
legal attention in the past few years. Because of the advances in
medical technology and the growing likelihood of a lingering
death in cases involving terminally ill patients, there has been
substantial public debate about the role of the individual in
determining the time and manner of death. By virtue of the
collective impact of increased public opinion in this regard, the
law has responded in several different ways—and with varied
degrees of success—to the legal problems confronting the terminally ill patient and the involved health care provider. It is the
purpose of this paper to examine the nature and scope of these
problems and to look at three specific legal vehicles that have
been offered in response to these problems—living wills, antidysthanasia contracts, and right to die legislation.

Overview

As a preface to considering the above described legal vehicles in detail, it is appropriate to examine the concept of euthanasia, or "good death" as the term is derived from the Greek. The word may generally be defined as an affirmative act that hastens the death of another because of a merciful motive to alleviate pain and suffering. It has been used interchangeably with such phrases as the *right to die, mercy killing, death with dignity,* and *painless inducement of death* (9, p. 86; 2, p. 509). Because the word implies the performance of an affirmative act it has become somewhat controversial and is used in this writing primarily for the author's convenience.

There are three primary categories of euthanasia that, for our purposes, shall include both acts and omissions. They are: (1) an affirmative act designed to bring about death, such as the injection of air into a patient's veins; (2) a refusal to commence, or continue further, ordinary medical treatment required to maintain life; and (3) a refusal to commence or continue further "heroic" or "extraordinary" measures to maintain life (7, p. 467).

In the first instance, i.e., the specific affirmative act designed to bring about death, the law technically considers the act to be a homicide, just as one might affirmatively act to fatally shoot another person. As a practical matter, there is no Anglo-American case in which a physician has been convicted of murder or manslaughter for having killed to end the suffering of a patient. The only attempted prosecution in this regard took place in 1950 when a New Hampshire doctor was brought to trial for injecting air into the veins of his cancer-stricken patient. Even though he confessed the deed and the attending nurse testified at trial that the patient was still gasping when the doctor injected the air, the apparent motive of mercy prompted the jury to acquit Dr. Sander (3, p. 66).

Despite this decision, however, the law strictly prohibits affirmative and intentional acts that are calculated to cause the death of another, regardless of the physical or mental state of the person performing the deed and without consideration of whether there may have been a valid consent to the action. The potential risk of criminal and civil liability in these situations is therefore clear and extreme (11, p. 142).

The legal picture blurs considerably, however, as one moves toward consideration of acts or omissions that fall within the latter two categories of euthanasia as previously described. In the second category of euthanasia, i.e., the withholding of ordinary medical treatment required to maintain life, one is concerned with treatment that falls plainly within the medical "standard of care" as recognized by the average well-qualified physician—treatment that may be considered typical, reasonable, or prudent. Generally, the law states that where a physician-patient relationship exists, there is a reliance on the part of the patient and a duty on the part of the physician that the physician will act to care for the patient in a competent and complete manner. Should the physician render treatment that falls below the applicable standard of care, it is done at the physician's legal peril. However, it is clear that before a physician may treat the patient there must be an authorization or informed consent. What is the physician to do if the proposed form of ordinary treatment for a given malaise is essential to the maintenance of the patient's life but the patient either refuses to give consent or is unable to give consent? This question has been addressed in a number of courts over the past decade with rather perplexing and contradictory results.

In a 1964 federal court case in Washington, D.C., *Application of President and Directors of Georgetown College,* 331 F.2d 1000 (1964), a federal judge refused to permit a woman to object to blood transfusions on religious grounds when transfusions were necessary to treat massive internal bleeding caused by a ruptured peptic ulcer. Among other things, the court referenced the need to protect the woman's 3-month-old child in refusing to allow the woman to choose to go to her death.

In a 1965 decision of a Connecticut federal court, *U.S. v. George,* 239 F.Supp. 752 (1965), a father of four minor children was ordered to accept blood transfusions against his religious objections on the grounds that the state had an interest in protecting the minor children and in upholding respect for the doctor's ethical conscience and professional oath that required him to treat the patient's condition.

In a 1971 New Jersey case, *John F. Kennedy Memorial Hospital v. Heston,* 58 N.J. 576, 279 A.2d 670 (1971), it was held that a patient could not refuse blood transfusions on religious grounds as the choice was equivalent to suicide and there existed no constitutional right to die. This case generally followed an earlier New Jersey decision, *Raliegh Fitkin-Paul Morgan Memorial Hospital v. Anderson*, 42 N.J. 421, 201 A.2d 537 (1964), where a woman in her 32nd week of pregnancy was precluded from refusing transfusions because of the state's duty to protect the life of the quickened fetus. And, in a 1965 New York case, *Powell v. Columbia-Presbyterian Medical Center*, 49 Misc.2d 215, 267 N.Y.S.2d 450 (1965), where a woman refused blood transfusions on religious grounds, the court held that it simply did not believe the woman meant what she was saying and concluded that, in fact, she must have wanted the transfusion. It was therefore ordered.

In 1965, the Supreme Court of Illinois in *In Re Estate of Brooks*, 32 Ill.2d 361, 205 N.E.2d 435 (1965), reversed a lower court decision, holding that the lower court's order requiring that blood be transfused into a competent Jehovah's Witness with no minor children and over her religious objection violated her constitutional right of freedom of religion.

The 1971 decision of a U.S. Federal Court of Appeals in *Winters v. Miller*, 446 F.2d 65 (1972) held that a hospital had to respect the wishes of a 59-year-old Christian Scientist who refused administration of medication. And, in the 1972 decision of *In Re Osborne*, 294 A.2d 372 (D.C. App. 1972), the court held that a 34-year-old man who, with full understanding of the facts of his situation, made provision for the support of his two children and executed a statement releasing the hospital from civil liability, could not be required to receive a blood transfusion over religious objection. Again in 1972, in the case of *In Re Raasch*, No. 455-996 (Milwaukee County Ct. Probate Div. Jan. 25, 1972) a Wisconsin court held that a 77-year-old woman could refuse to have her gangrenous leg amputated even in the absence of a religious basis for the decision. The judge ruled that a conscious adult who is mentally competent has the right to refuse medical treatment even when the best medical opinion deems such treatment necessary to save the patient's life.

Obviously, the case law relative to a refusal to commence or continue further ordinary medical treatment is unclear and of significantly minimal guidance in affording either guidelines or worthwhile protection to the physician or health care facility faced with such a medical-legal dilemma. Legal commentators have consistently stated, therefore, that having once undertaken the care of a patient, the physician or other health care provider is under a duty to render to the patient all ordinary care deemed reasonably necessary for the physical welfare of the patient. And, any inconsistent action creates substantial potential for liability.

In the final category of euthanasia—that of refusing to commence or continue further extraordinary care—it is the general consensus of legal writers that if such care is necessary merely to prolong life without expectation of success or benefit, such as artificially maintaining certain bodily functions of the individual that have no independent viability and without hope of returning the patient to health, it may be rejected by the competent patient without exposing the physician to liability for adherence to the patient's request. While the consensus of opinion seems to represent a reasonably clear legal theory, in practice the "extraordinary measures" cases present numerous legal problems.

Confusion exists as to the applicable standard for determining whether a patient is competent, especially when dealing with a patient who is terminally ill. There are further questions relating to the appropriate or relevant definition of extraordinary or heroic measures and to the standard of medical care that is to be applied to a patient in particular circumstances. Obviously, these questions can only be dealt with and answered by the courts. Unfortunately, however, there is a dearth of judicial precedent in this important area of the law.

Because of the legal quagmire surrounding medical decision making in the care of terminally ill persons, three legal devices of differing validity have been propounded to mitigate confusion of legal issues and concern for legal risks that have hampered clinical medical judgment in dealing with the right of the terminally ill patient to die with dignity.

The Living Will

The living will is a document used by competent adults who do not want to be kept alive by ordinary, extraordinary, or heroic measures if there is no reasonable expectation of recovery. It is drafted to resemble the same form of testamentary document that has been used since time immemorial for controlling the disposition of one's property at the time of death. The document is typically notarized or attested by at least two persons who affirm that the author was of sound mind and memory and acted voluntarily when executing the document.

The living will stands as an advance disposition of a person's life, which directs the physician to cease affirmative treatment under certain conditions (13, p. 371). It is intended to apply to both the situation in which a person with a terminal disease lapses into the final state of an illness or in the situation in which a victim of a serious accident deteriorates into a state of indefinite vegetated animation. Proposed language for inclusion into such a document, as recommended by the Euthanasia Educational Council is as follows:

> Death is as much a reality as birth, growth, maturity and old age—it is the one certainty of life. If the time comes when I can no longer take part in decisions for my own future, let this statement stand as an expression of my wishes while I am still of sound mind. If the situation should arise in which there is no reasonable expectation of my recovery from physical or mental disability, I request that I be allowed to die and not be kept alive by artificial means or heroic measures. I do not fear death itself as much as the indignities of deterioration, dependence and hopeless pain. (12, p. 509)

The document serves as an indication that at the time it was executed, the patient made a competent decision to reject future medical care given the occurrence of certain circumstances. And, in requesting that the patient not be kept alive by artificial means or heroic measures the patient's execution of the document represents a competent refusal of extraordinary means of treatment, which is largely recognized by commentators and theologians as consistent with the patient's right of self-determination, even more so than the refusal of ordinary means of treatment (6, p. 46).

Although clearly serving to address the significant legal question of patient competency to refuse life-threatening medical treatment in a situation of terminal illness, the living will fails to address other legal problems that attend the delivery of medical care in these situations. As a will, the document serves to provide cogent evidence of the patient's intentions in a terminal situation. However, the document does not serve as a mandate to the administering physician or health care facility and therefore is neither legally binding nor enforceable against them. Because the language of the will tends to be ambiguous, for example, " . . . no reasonable expectation of recovery," or " . . . artificial means, heroic measures," etc., the document vests considerable discretion in the physician without setting a standard against which the physician can make proper judgments. By failing to set uniform standards the living will fails to afford the necessary protection to encourage compliance on the part of physicians and other health care providers. Even if skillfully drafted so as to provide for the necessary specificity in its directives, the question of revocation of the living will by a terminally ill patient or by a court appointed guardian raises certain concerns. The question becomes whether a potentially irrational revocation can be allowed to undermine a previous rational consent to the living will document. If such a revocation were valid, the patient's true intention to refuse life-sustaining treatment could be neutralized and the purpose and effect of the living will overcome. Yet, to ignore such a revocation might be to deny the terminally ill patient any occasion to undergo a change of mind, whether or not the patient is rational, simply because the patient may be considered irrational by the physician.

While there exist certain questions regarding the efficacy of a living will, there can be little doubt that the existence of such a document will aid in the ultimate outcome of a dispute regarding the course of medical treatment for a terminally ill patient. Once the courts or the legislatures have had an opportunity to consider the use of living wills in particular fact situations, there will exist a substantial legal basis upon which to be guided in the proper construction and implementation of such documents. For the present, however, even in the absence of a developing body of common law to provide guidance in this arena, the living will stands as a reasonable alternative in helping to provide a solution to the legal problems confronting both patient and health care provider in the situation of terminal illness.

The Antidysthanasia Contract

The term *antidysthanasia* has been generally defined to mean a failure to take positive action to prolong life. The antidysthanasia contract is a vehicle intended to create a binding contractual relationship between an individual and those who will be responsible for the care of that individual in the event of terminal illness. Unlike the living will, which is unenforceable against the health care provider, the antidysthanasia contract would arise in the context of or incidental to the physician-patient relationship and would be executed by the parties to the agreement, thereby providing a potentially enforceable mechanism for dealing with legal problems arising in the context of terminal illness (10, p. 738).

The language of the contract must provide a detailed indication of the patient's unequivocal intention that life shall not be prolonged by ordinary or extraordinary measures when death is imminent or inevitable. And the terms of the agreement must describe in detail the rights and responsibilities of the health care provider and the patient in the terminal situation, setting out with utmost precision the standards against which medical decisions and judgments will be made if and when the terminal event occurs.

The document must be attested and signed by two competent witnesses who will provide testimony pertaining to the capacity of the signatory at the time the contract is entered into and to the presence or absence of any undue influence. The document should also be executed by all identified parties prior to the final institutionalization of the patient. Such a prehospitalization agreement offers an opportunity for the physician or other health care provider to participate in the drafting of the agreement. The terms of the contract are thus fashioned after the needs of all concerned parties. Usually, prehospitalization contracts will be concluded long before the potential for incapacity to draft a contract arises by virtue of an existing terminal illness.

There exists, however, another option—the execution of a document that would represent a continuing offer of the patient to receive medical care at some future time only upon the subsequent acceptance of the conditions of that offer by the physician or other health care provider. Such a document would be signed only by the patient prior to final hospitalization and would not be tendered to the health care provider for execution until the time of hospitalization. The significant problem occurs, however, when at the time of desired hospitalization there is no health care provider willing to sign the proposed offer. It is therefore most desirable to use the prehospitalization antidysthanasia contract approach, securing advance executed contracts from more than one institution or physician in order to assure flexibility in the event of injury or sudden illness.

The antidysthanasia contract tends to address and resolve the issue of patient competency in terminal illness situations by requiring advance execution. The documents are potentially enforceable against signatory health care providers and set out mutually agreed upon parameters for use in medical decision making during the final hospitalization. Nevertheless, there are recognized problems with these agreements.

Antidysthanasia contracts only bind specific parties and are not broadly applicable. An antidysthanasia contract with Dr. X at Hospital Y would be of little significance if sudden and extreme illness or injury occurred to a person in a different state or country. In addition, an antidysthanasia contract that may clearly spell out the agreed-upon parameters for decision making in the terminal situation may be declared void as against public policy in a jurisdiction where the action or inaction contemplated is considered illegal or criminal. Even if the contract is not declared void for public policy, immunity for the health care provider from prosecution by survivors of the deceased would derive only from the contractual terms and from no other more broadly applicable legal doctrine or standard. If an action against a physician for wrongful death were commenced as a result of the physician's compliance with the terms of an antidysthanasia contract, the physician might well have a defensible position to advocate, but weak acceptability of the antidysthanasia contract concept might seriously impair such a defense, resulting in potential judgment against the physician.

As a practical matter, the perceived problems with antidysthanasia contracts should rarely materialize, particularly because of the extremely personal nature of the contractual relationship. It involves very few persons, all of whom are ordinarily acting in concert with one another. To this extent, the contract may well be used as a positive and constructive means of legally justifying antidysthanasia in a setting of terminal illness. Nevertheless, this contractual vehicle has not gained widespread acceptance. There are certain risks involved in its usage that the cautious health care provider is usually unwilling to assume. Thus, in the absence of recognition and acceptance of the antidysthanasia contract by the courts or by state legislatures, it represents only a moderately helpful alternative in dealing with problems confronting both patient and health care provider in the situation of terminal illness.

Right to Die Legislation

In response to the recognized legal problems surrounding medical decision making involving the care of terminally ill patients, the legislatures of numerous states have begun to take significant steps in resolving these problems through enactment of "right to die" statutes. These statutes are a direct result of the collective impact of public controversy on the issues of death with dignity and the right to die, as well as the extensive commentary of noteworthy authors regarding proposals such as the living will and the antidysthanasia contract. Clearly, right to die legislation represents the single most effective vehicle for resolving the legal turmoil surrounding medical decision making relative to terminally ill patients.

It was not until 1976 that California became the first state to enact legislation providing the means by which a person could direct a physician to withhold or withdraw life-sustaining procedures artificially prolonging the moment of death. Following the California motion, Arkansas, Idaho, Nevada, New Mexico, North Carolina, Oregon, and Texas enacted similar legislation. Bills are still pending in approximately 15 states and only 12 states have definitely acted against such legislation. Even in the states that have rejected the enactment of right to die legislation, there is cautious optimism regarding the potential for change of attitude on this matter given a positive demonstration of success in those states that have already passed such laws (1).

A review of the pertinent aspects of the California law, known as the "Natural Death Act," will serve as an indication of the typical legislative approach to this issue. Virtually all states having right to die legislation have enacted these laws against the background of the California statute with very few substantive changes.

The California law recognizes that adult persons have the fundamental right to control decisions relating to their own medical care, including the decision to have life sustaining procedures withheld and withdrawn in instances of a terminal condition. Because modern medical technology has made possible artificial prolongation of human life, the California legislature concluded that in the interest of protecting individual autonomy, such prolongation of life that may cause the patient loss of dignity and unnecessary pain and suffering, while providing no medical benefit to the patient, must be avoided. Recognizing the uncertainty in medicine and law as to the legality of terminating use or application of life-sustaining procedures, where the patient has voluntarily and in sound mind evidenced a desire that such procedures be withheld or withdrawn, the legislature recognized the right of adult persons to make a written directive instructing their physicians to withhold or withdraw life-sustaining procedures in the event of a terminal condition.

After carefully defining the numerous terms contained in the statute, including such terms as "terminal condition"[1] and "life-sustaining procedure"[2] (notably without using such vague

---

[1] "Terminal condition" means an incurable condition caused by injury, disease, or illness, which, regardless of the application of life-sustaining procedures, would within reasonable medical judgment produce death, and where the application of life-sustaining procedures serves only to postpone the moment of death of the patient.

[2] "Life-sustaining procedure" means any medical procedure or intervention that utilizes mechanical or other artificial means to sustain, restore, or supplant a vital function, which when applied to a qualified patient, would serve only to artificially prolong the moment of death and where, in the judgment of the attending physician, death is imminent whether or not such procedures are utilized. "Life-sustaining procedure" shall not include the administration of medication or the performance of any medical procedure deemed necessary to alleviate pain. Cal. Health and Safety Code §718 (c) (1976).

phrases as "ordinary, extraordinary, or heroic measures"), the
legislature set out a standard form "directive to physicians"
that clearly represents the heart of the legislation. Having been
adapted from various living wills and antidysthanasia contracts,
the directive represents a uniform method for permitting the
competent adult to express the intention to refuse life-sustaining
medical treatment when death is imminent and the patient is
unable to give directions. The directive is to be honored by
family and physicians as the final expression of the patient's
right to refuse medical or surgical treatment and to accept the
consequences of such refusal (8, p. 23).

Witnessed by two adult persons who declare the signatory
party to be of sound mind, the directive is valid for 5 years and
may be re-executed as often as needed. Women, however,
stipulate that the directive shall be suspended if they become
pregnant. If the patient is competent in the event of a terminal
condition, the law requires the physician to determine whether
the existing directive is in accord with the patient's wishes. The
physician must also check to insure that the directive was
executed in accordance with the statute. The directive can be
revoked at any time by the author without regard for competency by defacing, destroying, or cancelling the document or by
signing a written revocation or verbally expressing such a
revocation to the attending physician (4, p. 6).

Interesting enough, the bill provides that death resulting
from carrying out the directive does not represent a suicide,
thereby resolving potential problems in relation to enforcement
of insurance policies. Moreover, the law precludes insurance
companies from invalidating, modifying, or failing to issue life
insurance policies as a result of receiving information that an
individual has in fact executed a directive to a physician.

The most important provision in the law is the section that
relieves physicians, health facilities, and licensed health professionals from civil, criminal, or administrative liability for carrying out a directive or for acting under the direction of a
physician who is carrying out such a directive under the terms
of the statute. This section affords the necessary immunity that
encourages widespread acceptance and implementation of the
law (5, p. 76).

As previously indicated, the California law is representative of the typical legislative approach to the enactment of right to die statutes. These laws squarely address the problems that hamper implementation of living wills or antidysthanasia contracts as a primary approach to resolution of legal problems confronting the physician and the patient in instances of terminal illness. Right to die statutes set up legislatively recognized standards against which physicians and other health care providers may, without impunity, exercise appropriate clinical judgment in dealing with terminally ill patients.

Conclusion

There are numerous legal problems confronting the physician or other health care provider engaged in medical treatment of the terminally ill patient. The most significant problem, however, derives from the potential legal liability that may result from inappropriate exercise of clinical judgment as viewed by any of a number of concerned parties involved in the terminal experience.

In order to eliminate the potential for such liability, three legal vehicles of differing effectiveness have been advanced for consideration. Each represents a unique approach to resolving the legal problems that attend medical care of the terminally ill patient. Nevertheless, right to die legislation is clearly the superior vehicle for accomplishing this objective. Unfortunately, at the present time only a few states have enacted such statutes. In other states, therefore, the living will or the antidysthanasia contract can provide the only reasonable legal alternative. Despite this fact, it seems an appropriate prediction that as right to die statutes continue to be implemented successfully, all states will begin to take a uniform legislative approach to legal problems arising in the terminal situation to insure a patient's right to death with dignity.

References

1. American Medical Association, Legislative Department. Death with Dignity. *State Health Legislation Report*, 1977, *5*, 15.

2. Beattie, J. The right to life. *The New Zealand Law Journal*, 1975, *5*, 501.
3. Fletcher, G. Legal aspects of the decision not to prolong life. *Journal of the American Medical Association*, 1968, *203*, 65.
4. Garland, M. The right to die in California: Politics, legislation, and natural death. *Hastings Center Report*, 1976, *5*.
5. Kaplan, P. Euthanasia legislation: A survey and a model act. *American Journal of Law and Medicine*, 1976, *2*, 41.
6. Kutner, L. The living will—Coping with the historical event of death. *Baylor Law Review*, 1976, *27*, 39.
7. Meyers, D. W. The legal aspects of medical euthanasia. *Biological Science*, 1973, *23*, 467.
8. Mills, D. H. California's natural death act. *Journal of Legal Medicine*, 1977, *5*, 22.
9. Sharp, T. H., Jr., & Crofts, T. H., Jr. Death with dignity—The physician's civil liability. *Baylor Law Review*, 1975, *27*, 86.
10. Smyth, J. A. Antidysthanasia contracts: A proposal for legalizing death with dignity. *Baylor Law Review*, 1975, *27*, 738.
11. Steele, W. W., Jr., & Hill, B. A legislative proposal for a legal right to die. *Criminal Law Bulletin*, 1976, *12*, 140.
12. Strand, J. G. The "living will": The right to death with dignity. *Case Western Law Review*, 1976, *26*, 485.
13. Turner, J. C. Living wills—The need for legal recognition. *West Virginia Law Review*, 1976, *78*, 370.

Request reprints from Theodore LeBlang, Southern Illinois University School of Medicine, Springfield, Ill. 62708.

ANNOTATIONS

THE LITERATURE—ANNOTATED BIBLIOGRAPHY

Edited by

PARIMALA DESAI

Abrams, R. D. The patient with cancer—His changing pattern of communication. *New England Journal of Medicine,* 1966, *274*:317-322. The article discusses and differentiates a cancer patient's communication at the three stages of disease: initial, advancing, and terminal and illustrates detailed case studies.

Adams, M. A. A hospital play program: Helping children with serious illness. *American Journal of Orthopsychiatry,* 1976, *46*:416. This paper describes a play-therapy program designed to facilitate the feelings, enhance the sense of mastery, foster adaptive behavior, and increase cooperation with medical treatment.

Adelman, S. E. Dying patient: An unspoken dialogue. *New Physician,* 1971, *20*:706-708. Dialogue between old man who is dying of cancer with young doctor.

Alsofrom, J. 'Hospice' way of dying—At home with friends and family. *American Medical News,* 1977, *20*:7-9. Author feels that Americans need to find a new way to die within their health care system. A hospice is one approach in which a team steps in to take care of terminal patients.

Armstrong, M. E. Dying and death—And life experiences of loss and gain: A proposed theory. *Nursing Forum,* 1975, *14*:95-104. The author attempts here to relate the similarities between the known data concerning the grieving process with observations of experiences of loss and gain.

Balasegaram, M. Carcinoma of the periampullary region: A review of a personal series of 87 patients. *British Journal of Surgery,* 1976, *63*:532-537. A total of 87 patients with carcinoma of the periampullary region treated by the author are reviewed. The clinical presentation and investigations are reported. In most cases treatment can only be palliative. Various forms of treatment are discussed.

Barrell, L. M. Crisis intervention: Partnership in problem solving. *Nursing Clinics of North America,* 1974, *9*:5-14. A cancer patient may go through crises many times, starting with initial awareness of diagnosis. Knowledge of the nature of crisis and crisis intervention give the nurse a valuable tool for helping the person to live with cancer.

Benoliel, J. Q., & Crowley, D. *The patient in pain: New concepts.* Proceedings at the National Conference on Career Nursing, American Cancer Society, 1974. The authors explore what pain is and how it varies in individuals. Implications of pain in cancer, with emphasis on nursing assessment and management, are discussed.

Bivalec, L. M., & Berkman, J. Care of parent. *Nursing Clinics of North America,* 1976, *11*:109-113. When a child has cancer, the entire family is under great stress. Family involvement in hospital care of the child increases the child's sense of normalcy, allows the family a sense of coping, and eases transitions between care at home and in hospitals.

Black, Sr. K. Social isolation and the nursing process. *Nursing Clinics of North America,* 1973, *8*:575-586. Social isolation has consistently been identified as a usual concomitant of the diagnosis of cancer. The author presents a sound theoretical base for understanding social isolation and suggests helpful nursing interventions that consider the person's own lifestyle.

Blewett, L. J. To die at home. *American Journal of Nursing,* 1970, *70*:2602-2604. This case study is about a terminally ill patient who was helped by four inactive nurses. Together they helped the patient remain at home and spend her last few months with her family.

Buckingham, R. W. et al. Living with the dying: Use of the technique of participant observation. *Canadian Medical Association Journal,* 1976, *115*:1211-1215. Technique of participant observation is presented as one approach to assessing care of dying patients and needs of their families on a surgical ward and a palliative care unit.

Buehler, J. A. What contributes to hope in the cancer patient. *American Journal of Nursing,* 1973, *73*:1588-1591. This article covers principles of self-help that relate to the cancer patient and family groups.

Bunch, B., & Zahra, D. Dealing with death: The unlearned role. *American Journal of Nursing,* 1976, *76*:1486-1488. Death is one of the major life events for which we have not learned effective role behavior. Real behavior instead of role playing is suggested.

Caldwell, D., & Mishara, B. L. Research on attitudes of medical doctors toward the dying patient: A methodological problem. *Omega,* 1972, *3*:341-346. A research experience that indicates a general reluctance on the part of physicians to discuss their attitudes about death.

Care of the dying. *British Medical Journal,* 1973, *1*:29. Symposium held at the Royal College of Physicians on November 29, 1972, examines home care, continuing care, and role of social worker, nurses, and local government.

Cotter, Sr. Z. M. Institutional care of the terminally ill. *Hospital Progress,* 1971, *52*:42-48. Author stresses importance of two components of effective institutional care of dying can be achieved by charismatic leadership and caring community.

Craig, Y. Care of dying child. *Nursing Mirror,* 1973, *137*:14-16. Author says that in the terminal stages of an illness, we deal with close survivors of the patient. Informed crisis intervention might promote better mental and physical health.

Craven, J., & Wald, F. S. Hospice care for dying patients. *American Journal of Nursing*, 1975, *75*:1816-1822. What people need most when they are dying is relief from the distressing symptoms of their disease, the security of a caring environment, sustained expert care, and the assurance they and their family will not be abandoned.

Davidson, G. W. *Living with dying.* Minneapolis: Augsburg, 1975. An attempt to interpret clinical data about technical illness from the patient's perspective. Based on interviews with more than 600 critically and terminally ill patients, their families and friends, and the health care personnel who served them.

Davidson, G. W. The waiting vulture syndrome. In B. Schoenberg et al. (Eds.), *Bereavement: Its psychosocial aspects.* New York: Columbia University Press, 1975. A case history of a patient's family rejecting her for not dying "on time." Includes recommendations to staff for helping the patient and family overcome their alienation.

Dobihal, E. F., Jr. Talk or terminal? *Connecticut Medicine*, 1974, *38*:364-369. Author discusses Hospice, Inc., a nonprofit corporation in the state of Connecticut, and how they have planned and coordinated patient-family unit care for the terminally ill.

Downie, P. A. Psychotherapy and the care of the progressively ill patient. *Nursing Times*, 1973, *69*:892-893. Discussion about treatment method of paralyzed patients, such as joint mobility, maintaining remaining muscle power, and retaining some measures of independence.

Durlak, J. A. Measurement of the fear of death: An examination of some existing scales. *Journal of Clinical Psychology*, 1972, *28*:545-547. This study is an investigation of the concurrent validity of four different psychometric scales that assess fear and anxieties about death.

Evans, A. E. Practical care for the family of child with cancer. *Cancer*, 1975, *35*:871-875. This discussion covers suggestions of practical ways to provide help for families of children with cancer: physical facilities for children's day care and parents' overnight stays, financial support, and parent group therapy.

Flynn, E. D. What it means to battle cancer. *American Journal of Nursing*, 1977, *77*:261-262. A doctoral prepared nurse finds that experiencing metastatic cancer means entering a new world full of confusion and uncertainty.

Found, K. I. Dealing with death and dying through family centered care. *Nursing Clinics of North America*, 1972, *7*:53-64. Detailed discussions such as the meaning of loss, the need to cope with crisis, prevalent attitudes toward death, and recognition of the grieving process provide a substantial framework from which meaningful interventions can be formulated to assist children and parents in handling the stress of death and dying.

Fox, S. Death of a child. *Nursing Times,* 1972, *68*:1322-1323. Author discusses the most distressing aspect of death, that of children.

Freeman, L. Care of the dying patient. *Journal of Family Practice,* 1976, *3*:547-555. Family practice grand rounds about care of the dying patient. Doctors and other concerned co-workers discuss their sharing experiences as well as statistical data.

Freihofer, P. et al. Nursing behaviors in bereavement: An exploratory study. *Nursing Research,* 1976, *25*:332-337. An exploratory study of 25 pairs of terminally ill patients and their loved ones to determine nursing behaviors that offer greatest support, comfort, and ease of suffering to loved ones.

French, J., & Schwartz, D. R. Terminal care at home in two cultures. *American Journal of Nursing,* 1973, *73*:502-505. An observation of two distinctive Arizona cultures and home care of their terminally ill patients (one a Navajo Indian and the other a white woman).

Fulton, R. Death and dying: Some sociological aspects of terminal care. *Modern Medicine,* 1972, *40*:74-77. Symposium for nonpsychiatrist about some sociologic aspects of terminal care.

Galton, V. A. Cancer nursing at St. Christopher's Hospice. *Proceedings of the National Conference on Cancer Nursing.* Chicago: American Cancer Society, 1973. The matron of St. Christopher's Hospice gives a warm, compassionate account of patient needs in the last few weeks of life: "the precious human personal touch," superb symptom control, sensitivity to the patient's wants, acceptance of his condition, and the nearness of caring persons.

Gammage, S. L. Occupational therapist and terminal illness: Learning to cope with death. *American Journal of Occupational Therapy,* 1975, *30*:294-299. Reports the role of occupational therapists in assisting a dying client to relinquish occupational roles. In addition, functions of listening to, accepting, and understanding the feelings of the dying person, the family, and the medical staff are described.

George, M. M. Long-term care of the patient with cancer. *Nursing Clinics of North America,* 1973, *8*:623-631. Communication is one of the most delicate areas surrounding cancer. The nurse is urged to demonstrate by words and actions respect for patients and family members as unique individuals in order to facilitate their open expression of feelings and realistic but hopeful anticipation of the future.

Grady, M. Assessment of the behavioral scientist's role with the dying patient and family. *Military Medicine,* 1975, *140*:789-792. Author discusses role of the behavioral scientist in the treatment of clients and patients between diagnosis of terminal illness and death, significance of crisis intervention for the family, and a transactional perspective that facilitates therapeutic relationships.

Gustafson, E. Dying: The career of the nursing home patient. *Journal of Health and Social Behavior,* 1972, *13*:226-235. The experience of aged nursing home patients is analyzed in terms of the "career" format developed by Roth. The passage of time and events is broken up into units according to an informal timetable. The conclusion of the study has both theoretical and practical implications.

Gyulay, J. Care of the dying child. *Nursing Clinics of North America,* 1976, *11*:95-107. From stages of terminal illness, nursing care to family participation and needs are discussed in detail.

Gyulay, J. E., & Miles, M. S. The family with a terminally ill child. In D. P. Humovich, & M. A. Barnard (Eds.), *Family Health Care.* New York: McGraw-Hill, 1973. Nurses are urged to practice family-centered care to the child and family throughout the course of illness from diagnosis until weeks or months after the child's death in whatever setting he is found: clinic, school, community. A useful assessment tool deals with the family's unique background, problems, strengths, and individual manner of coping with the crisis.

Hampe, S. O. Needs of the grieving spouse in a hospital setting. *Nursing Research,* 1975, *24*:113-120. The interdependence of family members prescribes meeting the needs of the cancer patient without also meeting the needs of the family members. This study of spouses of dying patients gives us strong prescription suggestions for nursing intervention with a dying patient and family members.

Harker, B. L. Cancer and communication problems: A personal experience. *Psychiatry in Medicine,* 1972, *3*:163-171. A mental health professional who has since died from her cancer writes of the very special problems she found inherent in a cancer patient's communication. Specific suggestions are offered to the patient, the family and friends, and the helpers and professionals.

Hertzberg, L. J. Cancer and the dying patient. *American Journal of Psychiatry,* 1972, *128*:806-810. This psychiatrist sees one of his most important functions on a cancer ward as consultant to the nurses.

Heusinkveld, K. B. Cues to communication with the terminal cancer patient. *Nursing Forum,* 1972, *11*:105-113. Author gives some vivid cues to deal with terminal cancer patients and ways that nurses can assist the patient and family to make the transition from life to death as comfortable as possible.

Hinton, J. Talking with people about to die. *British Medical Journal,* 1974, *2*:25-27. Sixty patients receiving care for terminal cancer commented on their discussion with doctors and nurses.

Hockey, L. Dying at home. *Nursing Times,* 1976, *72*:324-325. This article stresses that it is much better if old people with long illness die at home rather than in strange surroundings.

Holden, C. Hospices: For the dying, relief from pain and fear. *Science,* 1976, *193*:389-391. Author complements Dr. Saunder's unique contribution to sound medical management of terminal cancer pain, which is the main goal at St. Christopher's.

Holford, J. M. Terminal Care. *Nursing Times,* 1973, *69*:113-115. A look at total management of the terminally ill patient at home as well as in the hospital.

Holmes, H. A., & Holmes, F. F. After ten years, what are the handicaps and life styles of children treated for cancer? *Clinical Pediatrics,* 1975, *14*:819–823. To have hope, patients, families, and professionals need to know what treatments bode for the patient's future. A total of 124 long-term survivors of childhood cancer were questioned about therapeutic approaches, lifestyles, and quality of life, with gratifying results.

How patients help each other. *American Journal of Nursing,* 1975, *75*:1354. A brief article tells the facts about Orville Kelly's national organization, "Make Today Count," in which cancer patients help each other.

Idea Forum. Cancer crisis fund makes home care possible. *Hospitals Journal of the American Hospital Association,* 1976, *50*:14–16. Although home is often the best place for a cancer patient to be, home health care is not covered in most payment plans. One community has found a solution to this problem.

Ingles, T. St. Christopher's Hospice. *Nursing Outlook,* 1974, *22*:759–763. Author discusses firsthand experiences at St. Christopher's Hospice in England, its services, and how the staff performs.

Jaffe, L., & Jaffe, A. Terminal cancer and the coda syndrome. *American Journal of Nursing,* 1976, *76*:1938–1940. With wit and humor a devoted couple comment on how they courageously faced expected death but had difficulty maintaining the intensity of their companionship when death failed to arrive on time.

Keywood, O. Care of the dying in their own home. *Nursing Times,* 1974, *70*:1516–1517. Author discusses care of the dying at home, role of family, and procedures for the prescription and administration of drugs.

Kikuchi, J. How the leukemic child chooses his confidant. *Canadian Nurse,* 1975, *71*:22–23. The child, or the adult, with a life-threatening illness, confides in persons who are sensitive enough to pick up indirect cues thrown out to test reactions.

Klagsbrun, S. C. Cancer, emotions, and nurses. *American Journal of Psychiatry,* 1970, *126*:1237–1244. "Life is suddenly being lived." A cancer research unit was reorganized to place much of the responsibility for care on the patient and the family. Normal living was encouraged. People who had taken to their beds as part of withdrawal now got up to enjoy meals in the community dining room. Functioning again on an adult level decreased their anxiety, depression, and feelings of being a burden. Not incidentally, the unit became a tremendously more popular place for nurses to work.

Klagsbrun, S. C. Communications in the treatment of cancer. *American Journal of Nursing,* 1971, *71*:944–948. A psychiatrist pleads for improved communication with cancer patients to meet their needs for control, coping, and sharing.

Klein, R. A crisis to grow on. *Cancer,* 1971, *28*:1660–1665. Perceiving breast cancer as a crisis in the life of patient and family, a social worker delineates the psychological tasks a breast cancer patient must perform and specifies crisis intervention techniques professionals may use to help her through the crisis period. Healthy resolution of the crisis insures better rehabilitation.

Kobrzycki, P. Dying with dignity at home. *American Journal of Nursing,* 1975, *75*:1312–1313. Story of a young man who was, through teaching and coordination, able to achieve his wish to live and die at home even though he needed complex care.

Koenig, R. Dying vs. well-being. In *Nursing Digest Focus on the Care of the Elderly,* Wakefield, Mass.: Contemporary Publishing, 1975. Patients with chronic fatal diseases do not so much approach their death, they encounter the loss of their lives as their disease progresses. As progressive functional losses redefine the person's activity level, it is often possible to offer realistic hope of symptom control and comfort.

Kohn, J. Hospice movement provides humane alternative for terminally ill patients. *Modern Health Care,* 1976, *6*:26–28. Author gives vivid picture of development of hospice movement and its care for terminally ill patients.

Krant, M. J. et al. The role of a hospital-based psychosocial unit in terminal cancer illness and bereavement. *Journal of Chronic Disease,* 1976, *29*:115–127. Changes in societal and health care delivery patterns have decreased the support structures available to dying persons and their families. Krant sees the hospital offering many services continuously from predeath through bereavement.

Kron, J. Design a better place to die. *New York,* 1976, *9*:43–49. The symbolic and practical use of space can create a therapeutic milieu for the dying patient and the family. The design of the New Haven Hospice building, both practical and symbolic, encompasses the entire philosophy of humane dying.

Kübler-Ross, Elisabeth. Hope and the dying patient. In B. Schoenberg et al. (Eds.), *Psychosocial Aspects of Terminal Care,* New York: Columbia University Press, 1972, pp. 221–226. The well-known pioneer in death and dying illustrates how hope has different meanings to different people and to the same people at different stages of disease progression.

Kutscher, A. H. Psychopharmacological and analgesic agents in the care of the dying patient: For what end? In I. Goldberg et al. (Eds.), *Psychopharmacological Agents for the Terminally Ill and Bereaved.* New York: Foundation of Thanatology, 1973. Dr. Kutscher relates the use of drugs to the entire philosophy of psychosocial care of the dying, advocating prudent use of psychopharmacological and analgesic agents to assure dignity to every life.

Lamerton, R. C. Need for hospices. *Nursing Times,* 1975, *71*:155–157. Most people would prefer to die at home, but if this is not possible, care in a hospice, which is organized to provide a whole system of terminal care, would seem to be the next best thing.

Lester, D. et al. Attitudes of nursing students and nursing faculty toward death. *Nursing Research,* 1974, *23*:50-53. An investigation of the attitudes toward death and dying of 128 undergraduates, 66 graduate nursing students, and 62 nursing faculty at a university school of nursing in New York State.

Levinson, P. Obstacles in the treatment of dying patients. *American Journal of Psychiatry,* 1975, *132*:28-32. Obstacles in the treatment of dying patients are described and illustrated by case histories; specific recommendations related to the care of the more difficult cases are made.

Liegner, L. M. St. Christopher's Hospice, 1974. Care of the dying patient. *Journal of the American Medical Association,* 1975, *234*:1047-1048. Excellent article about how St. Luke's Hospital established a hospice program after Dr. Saunders had lectured there.

Lipman, A. G. Drug therapy in terminally ill patients. *American Journal of Hospital Pharmacy,* 1975, *32*:270-276. The treatment of the major discomforting symptoms of degenerative diseases—pain, anxiety, nausea, vomiting, and depression—is reviewed. Also, use of phenothiazines, anticholinergic drugs, and corticosteroids is discussed.

Lord, E. A. My crisis with cancer. *American Journal of Nursing,* 1974, *74*:647-649. A cancer nurse's ordeal with the disease has helped her to give empathetic support to cancer patients.

Lutticken, C. A. et al. Attitudes of physical therapists toward death and terminal illness. *Physical Therapy,* 1974, *54*:226-232. A study of attitudes of 115 clinical physical therapists toward death and terminal illness, determined by a 3-part questionnaire.

MacVicar, M. G., & Archbold, P. A framework for family assessment in chronic illness. *Nursing Forum,* 1976, *15*:180-194. In community health nursing and in long-term illness, the family is the unit of care. The framework presented here is an excellent tool to assess functioning of a family unit living with cancer.

Madden, B. W. Rehabilitation: Principles, philosophy, practice. *Proceedings of the National Conference on Cancer Nursing.* American Cancer Society, 1974, pp. 87-93. Rehabilitation philosophy is perfectly suited to meeting the cancer patient's need to live as normally as possible for as long as possible, focusing on what one has and not on what one has lost.

Maddison, D., & Raphael, B. The family of the dying patient. In B. Schoenberg et al. (Eds.), *Psychological Aspects of Terminal Care.* New York: Columbia University Press, 1972, pp. 185-200. The response to a dying member is examined in terms of individual family members, the family as a group, and the family in its relationship to society. Considered are areas of conflict mobilization, defensive operations, role changes, possible professional interventions.

Malkin, S. Care of the terminally ill at home. *Canadian Medical Association Journal,* 1976, *115*:129-130. This is a brief report of the experience with one group of 47 terminally ill patients cared for at home by greater Vancouver hospitals, with special attention given to physical, emotional, and psychological care.

Managements of patients with terminal cancer (symp.). *Postgraduate Medicine*, 1970, 47:202-206. Presentation of a minister who talks about the spiritual needs of the terminally ill patient, and an attorney who considers the medicolegal aspects of treating a patient who is near death.

Mann, S. A. Coping with a child's fatal illness: A parent's dilemma. *Nursing Clinics of North America*, 1974, 9:81-87. A compassionate nurse brings order to the coping tasks of parents with dying children, and to ways nurses may help the process. She suggests that while the nurse cannot evade emotional pain, "the rewards of witnessing and experiencing the tremendous courage of parents will far outbalance the painful aspects of participation in this tragic life crisis."

Marks, M. J. B. The grieving patient and family. *American Journal of Nursing*, 1976, 76:1488-1491. A short article relates ways to help grieving patients and their families in the hospital.

Martinson, I. M. et al. Home care for the child. *American Journal of Nursing*, 1977, 77:1815-1817. A report on an investigation of home care for terminally ill children, based on 29 experiences, by a team from the University of Minnesota.

McCaffrey, M., & Hart, L. L. Undertreatment of acute pain with narcotics. *American Journal of Nursing*, 1976, 76:1586-1591. Specific pharmacologic information that serves as the basis for refuting the common practice of underuse of narcotics, and for urging effective and safe use of narcotics for relief of pain.

McCorkle, R. Effects of touch on seriously ill patients. *Nursing Research*, 1974, 23:125-132. Nonverbal communication has long been taught as a primary means of conveying caring and security to a very ill person. This study methodically examines the effects of touch on a seriously ill person's behavioral and physiological status and supports its use in indicating a nurse's caring.

McCorkle, R. The advanced cancer patient: How he will live—and die. *Nursing*, 1976, 6:46-49. The patient with advanced cancer needs nursing help in learning to live with the disease: to communicate effectively, to relieve physical and mental distress, and to assist the patient and family with plans for their future.

McNulty, B. J. St. Christopher's out patients. *American Journal of Nursing*, 1971, 71:2328-2330. At St. Christopher's, dying patients are given excellent care to make them as comfortable as possible. Dying in familiar surroundings is preferred and that is why St. Christopher's home care program made it possible to give the best of services at home.

McNulty, B. J. Domiciliary care of the dying—Some problems encountered. *Nursing Mirror*, 1973, 136:29-30. Article is the author's observation of

784 patients for the period October 1969 to October 1972. Author's task was to maintain continuity of care by linking up with the general practitioner and the domiciliary services.

McNulty, B. The problem of pain in the dying patient. *Queen's Nursing Journal*, 1973, *16*:152-161. Sister McNulty urges attention to the physical, emotional, and comfort needs of a patient in addition to careful use of adequate drug therapy. Her particular orientation is to the terminally ill cancer patient in the home.

McNulty, B. The nurse's contribution in terminal care. *Nursing Mirror*, 1974, *139*:59-61. The director of nursing for the home care service at St. Christopher's Hospice offers a warm personal account of the needs of the dying patient and the family and of the art of caring for them.

Melzack, R. et al. The Brompton mixture: Effects on pain in cancer patients. *Canadian Medical Association Journal*, 1976, *115*:125-129. The McGill-Melzack Pain Questionnaire offers a tool and vocabulary useful in pain assessment. This questionnaire measured pain relief in terminally ill cancer patients when given the hospice medication in a palliative care unit (PCU) and in two other hospital environments.

Milton, G. W. The nurse in a cancer ward. *Medical Journal of Australia*, 1975, *2*:911-913. The value of discussion groups is stressed in clarifying the problems facing nurses who manage patients suffering from cancer.

Moore, H. Community nursing care study: Nine months in the life of a cancer patient. *Nursing Times*, 1977, *73*:59-60. This is a case study of a patient who finds out that he has an extensive cancerous growth and feels not only physically, but also financially and socially, crippled.

Mount, B. M. The problem of caring for the dying in a general hospital: The palliative care unit as a possible solution. *Canadian Medical Association Journal*, 1976, *115*:119-121. Author feels that the general hospital as a setting for terminal care has disturbing deficiencies, particularly the medical, emotional, and spiritual need of the patients and their families are neglected. Consideration to improve the situation led to the opening of the palliative care unit at the Royal Victoria Hospital in Montreal.

Mount, B. et al. Use of the Brompton mixture in treating the chronic pain of malignant disease. *Canadian Medical Association Journal*, 1976, *115*:122-124. Experience in pain control at hospices has evolved a revolutionary new philosophy and method for control of chronic pain, very different from control of acute pain. The aim is not treatment of pain but its prevention. No longer must the patient dread the return of agonizing pain to legitimize a p.r.n. medication.

Nolan, T. Ritual and therapy. In B. Schoenberg et al. (Eds.), *Anticipatory Grief*. New York: Columbia University Press, 1974, pp. 358-364. Reverend Nolan, who is also a registered nurse, believes that religious ritual has a therapeutic effect on cancer patients and their families in coping with anticipatory grief.

Northrup, F. C. The dying child. *American Journal of Nursing,* 1974, *74:*1066-1068. Communication is the ultimate goal when caring for a dying child, but this can occur only after comfort and caring needs are met.

Optimum care for hopelessly ill patients. A report of the clinical care committee of the Massachusetts General Hospital. *New England Journal of Medicine,* 1976, *295:*362-364. A report of the clinical care committee of the Massachusetts General Hospital, about how best to manage hopelessly ill patients.

Paige, R. L., & Looney, J. F. Hospice care for the adult. *American Journal of Nursing,* 1977, 77:1812-1815. The authors, clinical specialists for the Hospice project of St. Luke's Hospital Center in New York City, describe the integration of a hospice team within a hospital medical center.

Pain and suffering—A special supplement. *American Journal of Nursing,* 1974, *74:*491-520. A series of related articles about many new techniques of relieving pain.

Parkes, C. M. *Bereavement: Studies of Grief in Adult Life.* New York: International Universities Press, 1972. Ways in which people react to the experience of loss and grief provide a key to the understanding of human behavior in many situations of stress or crisis.

Parkes, C. M. Determinants of outcome following bereavement. *Omega,* 1975, *6:*303-323. The most serious of life changes carrying a health risk is death of a spouse. Parkes' studies of the bereaved identify factors that can alert us to the possibility of poor progress for survival.

Parkes, C. M. The emotional impact of cancer on patients and their families. *Journal of Laryngology and Otology,* 1975, *89:*1271-1279. A distinguished physician, long associated with St. Christopher's Hospice, examines psychosocial transitions and phases inherent in living with cancer and grieving over impending loss, both for the patient and the family.

Parsell, S., & Tagliarenia, E. M. Cancer patients help each other. *American Journal of Nursing,* 1974, 74:650-651. A self-help group for cancer patients initiated by a medical center serves the useful purpose of letting people know that they are not alone. The consistent themes that run through the meetings are helplessness, life and death, and the problems of everyday living.

Pattison, E. M. Help in the dying process. In S. Aretia (Ed.), *American Handbook of Psychiatry (Vol. 1).* New York: Basic, 1974, pp. 685-700. Refuting the idea that there is never a "nothing more to do" stage of dying, Pattison defines the fears of the patients and their families in coping with anticipatory grief.

Pellman, D. R. Learning to live with dying. *The New York Times Magazine,* 44f, December 5, 1976. To combat the isolation imposed by changed social and communication patterns sequential to cancer diagnosis, patients and families living with cancer are forming self-help groups to support each other. "Make Today Count" is one such group.

Pienschke, Sr. D. Guardedness or openness on the cancer unit. *Nursing Research*, 1973, 22:484–490. A study of the manner in which cancer patients were told their diagnoses and prognoses showed effects on patients' response to illness and to treatment.

Plumb, M. M., & Holland, J. Cancer in adolescents: The symptom is the thing. In B. Schoenberg et al. (Eds.), *Anticipatory Grief*. New York: Columbia University Press, 1974. Adolescents, involved as they are in the developmental transition from childhood to adulthood, respond to living with cancer—or dying from it—in special ways. Such realities as being "different" from their peers have meanings unique to this age group.

Proceedings of the National Conference on Cancer Nursing. American Cancer Society, 1974. A total of 35 papers presented at a September 1973 conference in Chicago focus many perspectives on how to help the cancer patient, child or adult, to live with cancer at home or in the hospital. A Professional Education Publication available from the American Cancer Society.

Proulx, J. R. Ministering to the Dying: A joint pastoral and nursing effort. *Hospital Progress*, 1975, 56:62–63. Author suggests that both chaplains and nurses should alter their traditional perspectives, the former by lowering their gazes from ethereal regions and the latter by raising their eyes from the mere physical. Where these lines of vision meet is the focal point of a new relationship between two key members of the health care team.

Purtilo, R. B. Don't mention it: The physical therapist in a death denying society. *Physical Therapy*, 1972, 52:1031–1035. Problems of terminal patients are outlined and practical guidelines are provided for the physical therapist.

Purtilo, R. B. Similarities in patient response to chronic and terminal illness. *Physical Therapy*, 1976, 56:279–284. Physical therapists sometimes hesitate to treat terminally ill patients. The author explains some important similarities in patient reactions to chronic and terminal illness. A conceptual framework of "little deaths" is presented for comparing the two types of illness.

Raft, D. How to help the patient who is dying. *American Family Physician*, 1973, 7:112–115. Author feels that a physician can help the patient who is dying by managing the patient's fear of pain and abandonment, denial of dying, anger and depression, and family acceptance of death through assurance.

Rees, W. D. Distress of dying. *Nursing Times*, 1972, 68:1479–1480. Comparative study of the patient dying at home and hospital. Various degrees of pain and distress charted during study.

Ryder, C. F. et al. Terminal care—Issues and alternatives. *Public Health Reports*, 1977, 92:20–29. Detailed discussion about issues and alternatives of terminal care in our changing society, professional attitudes, different concepts, and models of caring.

Saunders, C. A therapeutic community: St. Christopher's Hospice. In B. Schoenberg et al. (Eds.), *Psychosocial Aspects of Terminal Care*. New York: Columbia University Press, 1972, pp. 275–289. The Hospice's well-known medical director comments on dying at St. Christopher's. Uses illustrative photographs.

Saunders, C. Care of the dying. *Nursing Times*, 1976, *72*:1089–1091, 1133–1135, 1172–1174, 1203–1205, 1247–1249. Series of articles on care of the dying written by the well-known expert concerning nursing of patients.

Schultz, R. Meeting the three major needs of the dying patient. *Geriatrics*, 1976, *31*:132. Major three needs of the dying patient: control of paint, preservation of dignity, and love and affection discussed in detail.

Seldon, E. Even the elderly. *RN*, 1976, *39*:66. A story of the couple who managed their final days. A few days in their dream home helped this couple cope with death.

Share, L. Family communication in the crisis of a child's fatal illness: A literature review and analysis. *Omega*, 1972, *3*:187–210. A large body of literature is examined in relation to the protective approach or the open approach to the ill child in family communications.

Shneidman, E. S. Death work and stages of dying. In E. S. Shneidman (Ed.), *Death: Current Perspectives*. Palo Alto: Mayfield, 1976, pp. 443–451. Death work involves preparing oneself for death and for leaving loved ones. Shneidman, unlike Kübler-Ross, has seen not stages of dying but a clustering of intellectual and affective states set against a person's philosophy of life.

Shusterman, L. R. Death and dying: A critical review of the literature. *Nursing Outlook*, 1973, *21*:465–471. This is a survey of the major research projects primarily concerned with the experience of dying in a modern general hospital and gives special attention to the methodology that has been employed.

Stewart, B. M. Living with cancer. *Nursing Forum*, 1974, *13*:52–58. A nurse practitioner whose specialty is people, not tumors, applies her philosophy of health and of nursing to helping cancer patients repattern their lives into harmony with their environments, rather than patterning patients through a course of dying.

Stuetzer, C. et al. Mothers as volunteers in an oncology clinic. *Journal of Pediatrics*, 1976, *89*:847–848. Mothers of children who had died of cancer are serving as volunteers in a pediatric oncology clinic to improve communications, to alleviate frustrations, and to give emotional support to patients and their families.

Terminally ill patients welcome discussion in group counseling. *Geriatrics*, 1974, *29*:30. A short article about how a psychiatrist at Stanford University School of Medicine in California started a small-group counseling program for dying patients.

Vachon, M. L. S., & Lyall, W. A. L. Applying psychiatric techniques to patients with cancer. *Hospital and Community Psychiatry*, 1976, 27:582-584. Cancer patients live with the stigma of others' fears: that the patient is contagious, radioactive, or dying. Facing these difficulties and others associated with the response to cancer is facilitated in a Toronto hospital by weekly group meetings of patients, family members, and mental health staff.

Van Eys, J. Supportive care for the child with cancer. *Pediatric Clinics of North America*, 1976, 28:215-224. The "dying" child may live. Will she be developmentally sound?

Waechter, E. H. Children's awareness of fatal illness. *American Journal of Nursing*, 1971, 71:1168-1172. Author discusses the fact that terminally ill children "protected" by adult silence about their condition, may not express directly their awareness of and fears about their illness, but given the opportunity to do so indirectly, they will communicate their fears.

Wahl, C. W. Helping the dying patient and his family. *Journal of Pastoral Care*, 1972, 26:93-98. A psychiatrist suggests that refuting some of the erroneous beliefs terminally ill patients and their families have about dying may be one of the most valuable contributions made by various members of the care team.

Ward, A. W. M. Impact of a special unit for terminal care. *Social Science and Medicine*, 1976, 10:373-376. The impact study of a special unit for terminal care at Sheffield, England and how it has been accepted in the total system of care.

Weisman, A. D. On dying and denying: A psychiatric study of terminality. New York: Behavioral Publications, 1972. This in-depth study shows "denial" to be a complex phenomenon relating to a patient's perceptions of the primary facts of illness, the extensions and implications of illness, and death itself. Case studies illustrate throughout.

Weist, V. A. St. Christopher's Hospice. *International Nursing Review*, 1967, 14:38. Author gives account of how St. Christopher's Hospice was founded to be a home planned to allow patients to die quietly and happily.

Wentzel, K. B. The dying are the living. *American Journal of Nursing*, 1976, 76:956-957. Author stresses that dying patients need more attention, that there is a tendency to isolate them that runs completely counter to their growing need for companionship. At St. Christopher's Hospice in London, every terminal patient is treated individually with dignity and attention.

Whitman, H. H., & Lukes, S. J. Behavior modification for terminally ill patients. *American Journal of Nursing*, 1975, 75:98-101. Author discusses use of behavior modification techniques when the preterminal of terminally ill patient becomes a problem to self, family, and nurses.

Wilkes, E. How to provide effective home care for the terminally ill. *Geriatrics*, 1973, 28:93-96. A British physician gives specific suggestions for managing problems in home care. Yogurt for control of wound odor is one example.

Wilkes, E. Terminal care and the special nursing unit. *Nursing Times,* 1975, *71*:57–59. Author feels that because terminal care proceeds at such a slow pace for the majority of patients, the patient's emotional needs may be greater than routine nursing addresses. Special terminal care units, largely following the lead given over the years by Dr. Saunders at St. Christopher's, are suggested.

Witzel, L. Behavior of the dying patient. *British Medical Journal,* 1975, *2*:81–82. Study of 110 dying patients 24 hours before death, and 250 patients during weeks before death. Results are that 60 percent were well oriented as to time and space 24 hours before death and 26 percent were well oriented 15 minutes before death.

Yalom, I. D., & Greaves, C. Group therapy with the terminally ill. *American Journal of Psychiatry,* 1977, *134*:396–400. The authors describe their 4-year experiences with a therapy group for patients with metastatic carcinoma, helped by helping one another, by moving out of a morbid self-absorption, and by finding that they have much of value to share and to teach each other.

Yeaworth, R. C. et al. Attitudes of nursing students toward the dying patient. *Nursing Research,* 1974, *23*:20–24. A questionnaire to measure attitudes toward death and dying was administered to 108 freshman and 69 seniors in a baccalaureate nursing program.

Zinner, E. S. A proposal: Developing the role of clinical associates in the field of terminal patient care. *Journal of Thanatology,* 1971, *1*:156. This proposal was developed by a graduate student. Specifically, it proposes development of a new role in the health care field designed to aid the terminally ill patient in understanding and accepting the prognosis.

∞∞ ∞∞

THE MEDIA

∞∞ ∞∞

Reviewed by

Richard Dayringer

Southern Illinois University School of Medicine
Springfield

How I Use Audiovisual Materials.

Audiovisual materials add a great deal of interest for a class or seminar on any subject. They usually get participants much more involved in the subject and thereby encourage discussion. I try to introduce audiovisual materials with a statement about the topic to be addressed, some questions that should be faced, and some relevant facts and figures that may illustrate the issues in a direct way. I try to create interest by mentioning prominent scenes to be viewed.

I usually suggest that the audience pretend they are related to the main character of the film in their own professional role of doctor, nurse, pastor, etc. After the audiovisual is presented, I observe the effect on the group and first try to deal with their emotions by asking questions about their feelings. After dealing with their emotions clinically, I move on to the more academic or intellectual content to be discussed. I go with the discussion topics and try to feed in information that I want to disperse when I respond to questions, comments, and observations that are made. I also encourage participants to talk to or deal with one another's questions. The audiovisuals that I have reviewed in the following pages would fit nicely into a seminar on changing treatment concepts for the terminally ill and their families.

The first film, *How Could I not Be among You,* is primarily about one man's struggle with dying. This film could be used to deal with multiple issues individuals need to discuss in such a seminar. The poetry contained in the film is also available in book form and would be useful in the discussion to help people express feelings that they have as they identify with Ted and fantasize how they would feel if they were dying.

The second film, *Death,* presented the approach to dying patients in the 1960s. This could easily lead to a discussion of recent changes in the treatment of the terminally ill.

The third film, *The Dignity of Death,* depicts the first hospice. Its institutional concepts and philosophies and their transferability to North America could be discussed. Another discussion theme might address the difficulty institutions have in changing treatment philosophies and behaviors.

The two videotapes present the most recent treatment philosophy in this country. Patients are kept pain free with the use of morphine compounds. If the ethical issues involved in whether such medications should be used with the dying have not come into discussion, they could at this point. The advantages and problems of caring for patients at home could also be discussed after viewing these videotapes. Cost factors are another important topic.

In using audiovisuals along with a discussion period, summaries and conclusions become important. I think it would be most helpful for the seminar leader to write goals for each discussion and keep them well in mind so that he or she can draw conclusions and summary statements from the discussions.

Films

HOW COULD I NOT BE AMONG YOU?   *Thomas Reichman,* Eccentric Circle Cinema Workshop, Box 1481, Evanston, Ill. 60204. 30 min. color, 1970.

Tom Reichman has made a visual accompaniment for the writings of poet Ted Rosenthal, who at 30 learned he had leukemia. In free verse and awkward prose, Rosenthal expresses his reactions and shares his philosophy. There is much to absorb and the film can be viewed with profit more than once. The film is a song of dying. Its message is to live and love while you can.

Rosenthal responds to his prognosis with an intensified appreciation of the people and places around him. The terminal diagnosis releases him from previous cares. He feels free and unafraid. As his illness proceeds he describes his symptoms stoically but finally admits that he is "sick of dying" and that it is a "waste of time."

The film is well done; it is artistic and aesthetic. The language of the poet is emotional and "gutsy" enough to perhaps offend some viewers. After all, he was not working with a pleasant subject.

DEATH   *Arthur Barron,* Filmakers Library, Inc., 290 W. End Avenue, New York, N.Y. 10023.
40 min. black and white, 1968

This film is a documentary originally produced for NET in 1968 and is still a useful record. The staff of Calvary Hospital in the Bronx, New York, presents the problem of caring for the dying cancer patient.

The film opens with a hospital congregation at mass, singing in the chapel. This is the happiest scene in the entire film. In the next scene a physician states that the medical profession does not really know how to handle the terminally ill and as a result such patients tend to get isolated in a hospital—like Cavalry—that is willing to take them. There are a number of shots of patients being interviewed by members of the health care teams. All these patients speak of their excruciating pain and look as though they surely feel it.

One doctor kids the patients as he makes his rounds. "All right, everybody up!" "Why don't you people talk to each other in this ward? I think we ought to get rid of that TV."

The staff is shown in a seminar on dying where they discuss their own feelings and experiences with death and grief. In the orientation of new employees, they are told not to plan to cure the patients, but to care for them and make them comfortable. Patients are asked what advice they would give to new employees.

In one vignette a new aide insists that a patient looks all right when he is in pain and emaciated. He finally says, "Yeah, it's a great life." Later, he is shown being pronounced dead, wrapped in sheets and wheeled to the morgue while staff guards the halls to make sure no patients see this.

The last part of the film deals with a 52-year-old single man, Albro Pearsall. He tells his reaction to the care he has been given in the hospital. Albro's brother and sister-in-law share their views of what his life has meant. He complains of memory loss, weakness, pain, and loss of appetite. Home movie clips and snapshots of earlier, healthier times include family get-togethers, Albro in his Coast Guard uniform, and his apartment and keepsakes.

His former employer describes his work as excellent even though he was a loner. Albro describes himself as meticulous and seems to regret time spent in housework instead of outside activities. His employer remarks that "thousands leave no mark." But Mr. Pearsall has left an indelible mark through this movie.

He said, "All I am interested in now is relief from pain." In a visit with the chaplain, Albro says he has asked the Lord to take the pain from his body. His deathbed is also depicted along with his trip to the morgue and the funeral home.

This film honestly portrays dying as it has usually been accomplished by patients everywhere and unfortunately still is in many places. The stark reality of pain, isolation, and desperation that is presented does not produce a pleasant experience for the viewer, but, nevertheless, one in which much can be learned about caring for the dying.

THE DIGNITY OF DEATH   *ABC News*, 1973.

The most noticeable recurring sound in this film about St. Christopher's Hospice in London is, strangely enough since the average patient admitted has one month to live, laughter. In the opening scene with a doctor and nurse at a patient's bedside, the laughter of all three claims one's attention. Then, like an air-filled ball that cannot be kept under water, it keeps bouncing up here and there throughout the film. St. Christopher's Hospice certainly appears to be a happy place.

Children also have an invading presence in the movie. George Watson, the narrator, states, "Visitors are welcome anytime; children are always welcome." St. Christopher's provides a nursery for the staff's children. These children, along with those who visit the patients, make a vital contribution to the atmosphere.

Hospice is a medieval word that meant a stopping place for travelers, according to Cicely Saunders, who founded St. Christopher's in 1967. In this case it is a stopping place for patients, families, and even for staff who sometimes come right out of their professional schools to settle some personal dilemmas about death. St. Christopher's mission is the "spiritual treatment and medical care of dying men and women." Its goal is to "combine the learning of science and the wisdom of religion to relieve physical pain and mental anguish of dying patients and their families."

The physical setting of the hospice is bright and airy. There are wards with each bed having a colorful curtain around it. The patient's personal additions of flowers, paintings, personal articles, and lounge chairs give a feeling of warmth. "An untidy ward is a good ward," says Dr. Saunders in reference to the clutter of the patient's personal belongings. The nurses themselves also add to this atmosphere by wearing aqua uniforms.

The Christian religion also plays an integral part in the activities of St. Christopher's. According to Dr. Saunders, "We have found community but also something beyond ourselves." There are scenes of a chapel service with communion being served, two patients in different interviews mentioning religion, and interviews with both the chaplain, the Reverend Philip Edwards, and the Reverend Ed Dobihal, who has started a hospice in New Haven. The chaplain notes that no religious pressure is put on anyone.

This film presents the hospice concept of caring for the dying patient in a most favorable light. Two significant areas of St. Christopher's barely receive mention, however. The use of diamorphine (heroin) for the relief of pain along with Dr. Saunder's philosophy of drug use which she calls "polypharmacy" should have been given more attention, along with the bereavement service of the hospice, which follows families for up to 18 months. Nevertheless, the film does provide a rather comprehensive glimpse of St. Christopher's Hospice in less than 30 minutes.

TERMINAL CANCER: The Hospice Approach to Pain Control (Part 1)
with *Sylvia A. Lack*, M.D., Medical Director of Hospice, Inc.,
New Haven, Conn.
19 min. color, videotape, NCME, Roche, 1977.

Of all patients with terminal cancer, 50 percent require analgesics to control pain; 40 percent have pain that is moderate to severe in intensity. Proper attention to the details of prescribing medications will assure that the patient remains both alert and free of pain. Dr. Lack shows the viewer how to do this in the videotape.

Since 1967, when Dr. Cicely Saunders established the first hospice in England, 25 more have come into existence in that country. The first hospice was begun in the United States in 1971 at New Haven. There are now approximately 40 groups planning hospice programs in this country, and more than 10 are already providing patient and family care.

"Pain and cancer are not synonomous," according to the narrator, Dr. Lack. She maintains an opinion based on studies in England that 50 percent of all cancer patients have no pain. She does admit, however, that pain is the dominant symptom associated with cancer. She states further that "terminal cancer pain is purposeless, chronic, generalized, and has no perceivable end."

Dr. Lack strongly recommends administering analgesics before pain recurs. The formula for successful pain control at Hospice, Inc., in New Haven is (1) regular administration, (2) adequate dosage, and (3) oral medication whenever possible. She explains that a psychological dependence occurs only if a patient experiences pain between doses. Many physicians prescribe pain medication "prn" (as needed). Dr. Lack feels that this has no place in caring for terminal patients who, once treatment begins, should never be allowed to feel their pain and thus have to ask for relief. In fact, dosages are normally reduced as patients grow more confident that their pain is being controlled. They also become more relaxed. Excerpts from interviews with three patients are interspersed throughout the tape to verify Dr. Lack's conclusions. By giving medications orally in cherry syrup, the pain of an injection is avoided. When injected medications are needed, the patient usually requires institutionalization.

"Brompton's mixture," the famous British liquid composed of heroin, cocaine, alcohol, syrup, and chloroform water is not used in New Haven. It is not needed. Instead they use various ratios of morphine or methadone and phenothiazines.

While this videotape will be most useful to physicians who treat the terminally ill, it is also quite informative for all those in the health care field who work with those dying of cancer. Much more detail about dosages is charted and explained in the videotape than has been attempted here. Yet, Dr. Lack emphasizes the importance that all staff who work around the cancer patient maintain a commitment that pain can and will be controlled. "No patient should want to die because of the pain being suffered."

TERMINAL CANCER: The Hospice Approach to the Family (Part 2)
with *Sylvia A. Lack*, M.D., Medical Director of Hospice, Inc.,
New Haven, Conn.
19 min. color, videotape, NCME, Roche, 1977.

Caring for terminally ill patients and their families is different from most patient care, it's "curiously satisfying," according to Dr. Lack, the narrator of this videotape. Brief segments of interviews with various members of one family by Dr. Lack, a social worker, and a nurse are inserted throughout to give credence to views being asserted.

The approach to families espoused is that taken by Hospice, Inc., which was funded in part by the National Cancer Institute.

The family is seen as the unit of care in terminal illness and is incorporated as part of the health care team. Hospice staff teach the family to care for the patient at home and to provide nursing care until readmission or death. Thus, the family can apply its hard-won knowledge of the patient's particular likes and dislikes. The family may prefer to hire someone to help with household work rather than a nurse if the family gives good nursing care. Patients and their families have available a continuous telephone service provided by the hospice. Families frequently test this at first to be sure it is there, but then their use of it diminishes.

Families are educated to budget their strength and finances with a terminal patient since things will get worse rather than better and easier. Admission to this hospice or a hospital, they are assured, doesn't mean that the family has failed, only that their patient's needs have changed. The hospice encourages families to be involved in the patient's care even during institutionalization. Dr. Lack believes that this reduces their guilt feelings at the time of death. Flexible visiting hours provide easy access to the patient, the presence of children (a sign of one's own mortality), permission to help care for the patient, and space for families such as a family room.

One thing puzzled me about this program. The purpose of the hospice was stated as follows: "to meet the physical, spiritual and emotional needs of patients and their families." Yet, no further word was uttered throughout this tape (or Part I of the series) about meeting the spiritual needs. No chaplain was pictured in any of the scenes.

This program should prove to be helpful, informative, and hopefully, mind-changing to physicians and those in adminsitrative positions. Nurses could learn much from it that would make their work easier and more interesting as well as allowing families to feel more useful. Social workers and chaplains should be able to support most of the suggestions.

Audiovisual Notes

A conference on the dying child. Barbara Brodie, Carol Alexander, Rosalie Belniak, Barbara Logue, 16 mm, 44 min, black and white, 1967. Presented are the problems of nurses' emotions in caring for the dying child, how they must accept them and the emotions of the family, how the child learns the concept of death, inadvertent changes in the care of the child who is dying, and how support might be given to child and parents alike.

A special kind of care. American Journal of Nursing, 16mm, 13 min, color, 1968. Demonstrates the emotional impact of a diagnosis of advanced cancer on a family.

Basic principles of terminal care, F. R. Gusterson, 28 min. Need for key manager for care of each patient and for communication; relationship with patient and family to gain confidence; control of pain; etc. Audience—GP's, junior hospital staff, nurses, Or. MRSF.

Care of the patient who is dying. Filmstrip, 35 mm, color (cassette/record) with instructor's guide. Trainex Corporation. Guides the learner to accept the events accompanying death in the hospital and to cope with the emotional reactions that occur in the hospital staff, the family, and the patient.

Care of the patient with terminal cancer. Filmstrip, 35 mm, color (cassette/record) with instructor's guide. Trainex Corporation. Focuses on many aspects of physical care and psychological support necessary for patients with terminal cancer.

Group therapy with a terminal patient. Videotape, 50 min. Produced by Walter Reed Army Medical Center, Washington, D.C. WR 109-5, Reel No. 61, 1975. This tape consists of an interview with a terminal patient concerning marital problems associated with a terminal illness and other psychosocial elements of treating the needs of the terminal patient.

Guidelines for interacting with the dying patient. Filmstrip, 35 mm, and 1 cassette, color (1/2-track mono. 22 min), 1972. Concept Media presents perspectives on dying—program 4.

Hazards and challenges in providing care. Filmstrip, color, 35 mm, and 1 cassette (1/2-track mono. 28 min). Concept Media presents perspectives on dying—program 3.

Just a little time. Barey-Callaci-Video Nursing, 16 mm, color, 21 min, 1973. Production made possible by a grant from the Samuel S. Fels Fund, Philadelphia, Pa. A documentary exploration of the shared experience of a 49-year-old terminally ill woman and her nurse, Mrs. Dona LeBlanc, a nurse specialist in oncology. The dialogue reveals the unique rewards as well as the special problems involved in the relationship between the nurse and the dying patient.

Just a little time. Barey-Callaci-Video Nursing, 1973. This audiocassette and study guide are designed to be used in conjunction with the film of the same title. The recording consists of a conference among nursing staff concerned with developing a plan of care for the patient in the film, a 49-year-old terminally ill woman.

Management of the terminally ill: The family. Network for Continuing Medical Education, VC 3/4 in, black and white, 16 min. Offers practical help to physicians in dealing with the dying patient.

Nursing management of the dying patient. American Cancer Society, 5" reel/cassette, 21 min. Points out the varied ways in which people perceive and react to their dying, and how each needs to be treated as an individual.

Religion and the clergy. Videorecording, University of Washington Health Sciences Learning Resources Center, 1 cassette, 35 min, black and white, 1974.

Terminal patients: Their attitudes and yours. 16 mm, 16 min, Abbott Laboratories, 1974. Explores staff attitudes toward caring for the terminally ill and probes the thoughts of two dying patients.

Till death do us part. Videotape, 55 min. Produced by Walter Reed Army Medical Center, Washington, D.C., WR 109-75, Reel No. 61, 1975. The tape depicts psychotherapy interviews with five terminal patients. The emphasis is both content- and process-oriented. This program demonstrates feelings, attitudes, and interpretations of patients undergoing treatment of cancer.

To take a hand. Motion picture, University of Texas, M.D. Anderson Hospital and Tumor Institute at Houston, 1 reel, 16 mm, 17 min, color, 1969.

A DIRECTORY OF HOSPICE PROGRAMS
IN THE UNITED STATES

Arizona

Hillhaven Hospice   *Sr. Teresa Marie, Administrator, 5504 East Pima,*
Tucson, AZ 85712 (602-886-8263)

Hillhaven is a nonprofit group under the Hillhaven Foundation and is scheduled to receive NCI funds. Patient care began in April 1977. The hospice is licensed as a skilled nursing facility. Care is provided continuously, either in the home, in a clinic at Tucson East Community Mental Health Center, or in their inpatient facility. No care is provided to children under 16, but they are negotiating for a special hospital license which will permit this. They are averaging 8 patients weekly at this time. The staff consists of seven registered nurses, four nurses aides, one physician, one social worker, one volunteer director, and five consultants. Collaboration with other service agencies takes place. The fee for services is determined on a sliding scale for home health care (nursing and counseling). Inpatient care is $55.00 per day, $60.00 per day for a private room, and $10.00 per day for day health care. Service area is 9,241 square miles, populated by 400,000 people. Volunteers are utilized and there are currently 45 available. The 39-bed facility was opened in 1977 and the major goals for the next 12 months are to further acquaint community physicians with the hospice concept, particularly pain control measures, obtain special hospital license, implement their own home health care program, and create a smooth, effective operation of the program.

California

Community Support Group-Hospice Concept   *Joan Parker, Secretary,*
21 Willow Road, Menlo Park, CA 94025

A nonprofit, not incorporated, group not providing patient care. A loosely affiliated group of doctors, nurses, social workers, clergy, health administrators, counselors, and volunteers, who represent a multiplicity of agencies and offices in the Peninsula Area, and who are interested in integrating aspects of hospice care into existing health care systems. Group meets monthly for continuing education, communication and moral support.

Compiled originally from a directory provided by Hospice, Inc., New Haven, and updated and corrected by each program director in December 1977.

Hospice of Marin   *Barbara Hill, Executive Director, William M. Lamers, Jr.,*
M.D., Medical Director, P.O. Box 72, Kentfield, CA 94904

This nonprofit group, incorporated in 1976, has provided outpatient care since December 1975. It is licensed as a home health agency. Care is provided continuously either at home or in an institution in Marin County. Services to children are provided and the average number of patients cared for weekly is 20. The staff includes five registered nurses, four physicians, five social workers, one volunteer director, and nine consultants. There is no fee for services. The service area numbers 200,000 in population and is 80 square miles in area. At least 26 volunteers participate, both lay and professional. Major sources of funding are contributions from friends and memorials, and several foundation grants.

Hospice of Santa Barbara, Inc.   *Sidney J. Smith, Executive Director,*
1525 State Street, Suite 11, Santa Barbara, CA 93101

A nonprofit group incorporated in December 1974 that provides patient care within the home and, on a limited basis, with an independent hospital palliative care unit and other care facilities. Services are provided to anyone regardless of age or financial status. At present, 45 persons are served. Care is provided in collaboration with other community service programs including visiting nurses, the county social service, and in consultation with the county medical society and pharmacologist organizations. No fee is charged. The service area is 3,000 square miles with a total population of approximately 225,000. Four chapters are located within the county, all under one administrative head. Both professional and nonprofessional volunteers are included in the outreach program, with approximately 50 persons involved. Educational programs for volunteers are held twice a year, with 100 people usually attending. A complete 7-week course of education is required of volunteers, plus a screening process and observed service situations prior to being placed in a home care situation on their own. Funding sources include a Presbyterian church grant, a grant from the area agency on aging, funding by the California Division of the American Cancer Society, plus support from city and county revenue sharing, and one CETA position. Additonal program potential to be developed and refined during the next 12-month period includes: "Long Term Patient Relationships," "Bereavement Needs," "Special Programs for Youth," and "Family Counseling."

Kaiser-Permanente Medical Care Program   *T. Hart Baker, M.D.,*
Regional Medical Director, Southern California Permanente Medical Group,
1505 Edgemont, Los Angeles, CA 90027

A nonprofit group that is officially part of the Kaiser-Permanente Medical Care Program. Patient care has yet to begin. Major source of funding is Kaiser-Permanente Medical Care Program and the National Cancer Institute. At the present time the hospice program is in the planning stage. Preparations are being made to negotiate with the National Cancer Institute for an award of a contract for a hospice demonstration program and evaluation. Plans call for beginning the hospice program in January 1978.

Parkwood Community Hospital   *Joseph A. Aponte, Administrator,*
7011 Shoup Avenue, Canoga Park, CA 91304 (213-348-0500)

The hospice is part of Parkwood Community Hospital—an acute care investor-owned facility providing patient care on half of a surgical unit separated from the main unit. Average number of inpatients cared for weekly is 5–8, outpatients average 10–15. Ancillary support and bereavement programs serve 80–100 people. The hospice collaborates with the American Cancer Society and local in-home health services and skilled nursing facilities. The staff includes registered and licensed practical nurses, physicians, and a clinical social worker. The service area is 150 square miles and has a population of 1.5 million. Major source of funding is derived from patient charges.

Colorado

Penrose Hospital   *2215 North Cascade Avenue, Colorado Springs,*
CO 80907, Mrs. James V. Carris, 1334 Culebra Avenue, Colorado Springs,
CO 80907 (303-475-2600)

One floor of the 372-bed, acute care, nonprofit, Catholic Penrose Hospital is set aside for treatment of cancer patients. Some hospice services are included in the total care of the patient and family. Four rooms are decorated in a homelike manner for patients and families to congregate, rest, eat, sleep, observe TV, and consult with physicians or clergy in privacy. Families and children may visit patients at any time. Volunteers serve on the floor to add supplementary care. There is a full-time oncology social worker and nurse practitioner. Pastoral care is part of the total hospital program. Two weekly sharing sessions are held, one for outpatients and families and one for inpatients and families. Home nursing is coordinated and provided through the Visiting Nurses' Association. A very modest effort is made in the area of bereavement counseling. Future expansion of the total care philosophy is under consideration for other floors in the hospital. The hospice philosophy of palliative treatment and attitude toward death will be extended to a satellite hospital if its acquisition materializes as planned.

Connecticut

Hospice, Inc.   *Dennis Rezendes, Executive Director,*
765 Prospect Street, New Haven, CT 06511

Incorporated in November 1971, this nonprofit organization has been providing patient care since March 1974. Licensed as a home health agency, over 380 patient/families have been served through their program. Land has been purchased and construction on a 44-bed inpatient facility will begin in Branford. Care is presently provided in the home. Funding has been through a contract with NCI that ended in 1977. At that time third party payment is expected to begin with fees for services previously free. Staff includes registered and licensed practical nurses, a social worker, physicians, and various consultants. Volunteers are utilized in home care and in office duties. Over 6,000 volunteer service hours were logged in 1976 by an average of 50 volunteers. The state of Connecticut has included $1.5 million in the current budget to help the hospice construct its new facility and the federal government has voted an additional $1 million for the same purpose.

District of Columbia

Washington Hospice Society, Inc.   *Sr. Mary Margaret Meldon, Executive Director, 1511 K Street, N.W., Washington, D.C. 20005 (202-638-1300)*

A nonprofit group incorporated in April 1977 not yet providing patient care. Task forces are organized. Original source of funding came from Washington Cathedral, and they have received subsequent funds ($15,000) from the American Cancer Society District of Columbia Division and individual donors. Immediate objectives include feasibility studies on freestanding versus non-freestanding facilities, ways of raising major funds, and need for home care programs in the area.

Florida

Hospice Orlando   *Daniel C. Hadlock, M.D., President of the Board and Medical Director, P.O. Box 8581, Orlando, FL 32806*

Has been functioning with patient care since October 1976 and has, as of December 1977, worked with over 126 patient/family units. It incorporated in April 1977 and has a functioning Board of Directors. In March 1977 they were awarded $1,000 for special health services, having applied through the Community Service Award program of Walt Disney World, and received a $2,000 grant from the American Cancer Society in September 1977. Volunteers are used in the program.

Georgia

Hospice Atlanta, Inc.   *Harry Hamil, Coordinator of the Board, 1055 McLynn Avenue, N.E., Atlanta, GA 30306 (404-875-6963)*

A nonprofit group, incorporated in November 1976, officially part of the Unitarian-Universalist Congregation of Atlanta. Home care is presently being provided, implementing an entirely volunteer organization. Major source of funding is through contributions. Major goals for the next 12-month period are (1) expansion of the home care program, (2) training volunteers, (3) completing a feasibility study for an inpatient facility, and (4) continuing a community information program.

Illinois

Highland Park Hospital   *Marge Lyons, R.N., Counselor, 718 Glenview Avenue, Highland Park, IL 60035*

Highland Park Hospital is a nonprofit hospital utilizing the wholistic patient care concept for all patients. Emphasis of the program is on meaningful, productive living in the face of life-threatening illness. Careful attention is given to symptom control, with extra nursing care provided as needed. Many community service agencies collaborate in this program. Highland Park Hospital is a 334-bed hospital serving an area on the north shore of Chicago. The program involves a varying number of specially trained staff, volunteers, and chaplains. The wholistic program at the hospital is funded by private donations and regular hospital fees. No additional charges are made to the patient for this care. Future plans involve expanding the program to bring support people to patients in their own homes. This goal is being achieved with the aid of visiting nurses, trained volunteer staff, and involvement of the area religious communities.

St. John's Hospital *James Cox, M.D., Chairman,*
Southern Illinois University School of Medicine, Department of
Family Practice, P. O. Box 3926, Springfield, IL 62708
(217-782-5872)

This group is officially part of St. John's Hospital. They are not providing patient care at this time. Volunteers are part of the planned program and a major source of funding has yet to be determined. A facility has been acquired and recruiting of a physician/director and head nurse is in process.

Maine

Hospice of Maine, Inc. *32 Thomas Street,*
Portland, ME 04102, (207-774-4417)

A nonprofit group that was incorporated in November 1976 and provides patient care through trained volunteers. Service began in November 1976. Care is provided at home, and on the average, three patients are cared for weekly. All staffing is done on a volunteer basis by the board of directors. Presently they are collaborating with other service agencies. No fee is charged for services. Major source of funding is from contributions and memorials. The service area numbers 250,000 in population and is 100 square miles in area. Eighteen volunteers are used and are supervised by the board of directors.

New Hampshire

The Salemhaven, Inc. *Rev. Daniel V. Weaver,*
8 Pleasant Street, Salem, NH 03079

A nonprofit, incorporated group. No patient care is presently provided. Currently processing HUD 232 programs to build 100 beds for nursing care, essentially as a nursing home. The hospice program will work within this framework and construction is planned for March 1978.

New Jersey

Overlook Hospital   *L. Stephen Hartford, Vice President–Ambulatory Services, 193 Morris Avenue, Summit, NJ 07901*

Overlook's hospice home care program was established in January 1977 as an extension of an existing home care department. Hospital staff with full-time assignments to the program include two registered nurses and a volunteer director. Other personnel assigned on a part-time basis include a physician, a chaplain, a social worker, a psychologist, a nutritionist, and an occupational therapist. Services purchased from other agencies include home health aides and equipment. The staff provides emotional support as well as physical care. A volunteer component scheduled to be implemented in January 1978. The service is available to patients with any type of terminal illness and to all age groups. The daily census has averaged 20 patients of whom the majority are over 65 and suffering from cancer. There is a fee for physical care services rendered, based upon cost and scaled according to ability to pay. Health insurance, especially Medicare, has been the major source of funds. Overlook is a 541-bed, nonprofit community/teaching hospital located in a suburban area of north-central New Jersey. The hospice home care program is limited to the 11 municipalities comprising the hospital's service area.

New York

Burke Rehabilitation Center   *Charlotte M. Hamill, Associate Director, 785 Mamaroneck Avenue, White Plains, NY 10605*

A nonprofit group not providing patient care at this time. Definition of program awaits development of plans for a skilled nursing facility.

Haven of Schenectady   *Mrs. Jeanette Neisuler, 2217 Niskayuna Drive, Schenectady, NY 12309*

Being formed.

Hospice Committee   *Ms. Nina McPhilmy, Chairman, RD 2, Box 96, Corning, NY 14830*

Being formed.

Hospice of Rockland, Inc.   *Joe Brass, Executive Director, 4 Union Road, Spring Valley, NY 10977*

Rockland is a nonprofit group incorporated in February 1977. It is an outgrowth of the Elaine Sanders Memorial Foundation, Inc. Patient care has been provided since

February 1977. Care is available continuously, depending on the situation. A physician is available for consultation and referrals at the hospice office. All services are coordinated with existing agencies and supplemented by 30 hospice volunteers. The volunteers include many people from the medical and social service professions. Affiliation with two hospitals has been arranged to care for inpatients when needed. All volunteers take a 10-week training program. At present there is no paid staff. Present case load averages about 20 patients per week. Individual and group counseling is available to the families. Services are available to children under age 16. There is no fee for services. The service area has a population of 287,000 people. Major source of funding is private contributions. Home care license and inpatient facility applications are presently pending and grants are being sought. During the next 12 months the director hopes to have a paid staff of professionals so that services may be expanded.

Hospice at St. Luke's   *Chaplain C. J. Sweetser, Chairman,*
Hospice Committee, St. Luke's Hospital Center, 114th Street and
Amsterdam Avenue, New York, NY 10025 (212-870-1732), or
(212-870-6775)

This program provides hospice care through a consulting team of health professionals associated with St. Luke's Hospital Center. Upon referral from physicians the team of nurses, social worker, chaplain, and physicians visit inpatients and family daily, providing expertise in symptom control. Outpatient services are coordinated with the certified Home Health Agency at St. Luke's as well as various community agencies. Outpatients are maintained by periodic visits to St. Luke's clinic and hospice team telephone calls and home visits. Care of patients and family includes bereavement follow-up. Costs for care are provided in two ways: in- and outpatient charges are assumed by third party reimbursement groups; hospice team salaries and adminstrative expenses are supported through private gifts and foundation grants. Patients are not charged for hospice consultant services. This program has been operational since April 1975, and provides services to referred patients, primarily in the 90,000 population catchement area of St. Luke's. The team consists of three clinical nursing specialists, one of whom is program coordinator, one social worker, three part-time physicians representing oncology and psychiatry, and one chaplain. Future plans include expansion of patient population, an organized training program for volunteers, and research studies.

Our Lady of Lourdes Memorial Hospital   *David M. Bloom, M.D.,*
169 Riverside Drive, Binghamton, NY 13905

A nonprofit, unincorporated group that operates as a part of Our Lady of Lourdes Memorial Hospital. Patient care began in December 1975 on a 24-hour basis. Services to children under 16 are provided. No fee is charged for services. Volunteers are not part of the program. Major source of funding is the hospital. Immediate goal is to apply to the New York State Department of Health for permission for in-hospital service and to establish home care.

North Carolina

Hospice of North Carolina, Inc.   *Carl L. Whitney, Executive Director,*
P.O. Box 11452, Winston-Salem, NC 27106

This nonprofit group was incorporated in April 1977 and has now been granted tax-exempt status by the IRS. The executive director is full-time. The statewide organization is an educational, training, and support group whose intent is to enable development of local chapters that will provide hospice care. Presently there are chapters, or interest groups, in Charlotte, Winston-Salem, Greensboro, Asheville, Raleigh-Durham-Chapel Hill, Greenville, and Wilmington. Home care in one or more of these locales is expected to be offered by the end of 1978.

Texas

Hospice of Southeast Texas   *The Rev. William Manger, President,*
312 Pine Street, Orange, TX 77630

A nonprofit group incorporated in December 1976, not now providing patient care. Funding is being sought from foundations, private individuals, groups, and organizations. Certification of need was submitted November 30, 1977. Services will start April 1, 1978 if granted. During the next 12-month period goals are to begin home visiting services, to obtain monies, and to receive a certificate of need for an inpatient facility.

Virginia

Haven of Northern Virginia, Inc.   *Dorothy N. Garrett, Coordinator,*
7300 McWhorter Place, Annandale, VA 22003 (703-941-7000)

A nonprofit group incorporated in February 1976. Care began in September 1976. Supportive and counseling care is provided where the patient and/or the family members are at any time. Age range: from birth to old age. The average number of patients (or families) is over 100 each week. More than 160 volunteers provide services. Volunteers include nonprofessional and professional. Professionals (physicians, psychiatrists, social workers, the clergy) work in supportive and consultant roles for the volunteers, and may be called in to offer expertise directly with patients as they see the need. Nurses do supportive, not primary, nursing care, at times working as the extension of Public Health and Visiting Nurses, and also offer home-care education to families as well as relieving primary care givers in the home for needed rest. Collaboration with several service agencies and hospitals takes place. No fee charged for services. The service area has a population of 850,000. Total volunteer organization with a coordinator, board of advisors, and board of directors. Major sources of funding are donations and a grant during 1977-1978. Long-range help has been given to more than 225 families since September 1976 with another 300 families receiving short-range help and follow-up. Individual help and group sessions are held every other week for widows and parents who have lost children. Groups for widowers, teens, and parents who have seriously ill or chronically ill children are being organized.

Wisconsin

Bellin Memorial Hospital   *Thomas R. Leicht, M.D., Medical Director, P.O. Box 1700, 744 South Webster Avenue, Green Bay, WI 54305*

Leadership is provided by Thomas Leicht, M.D., Kathryn Andrews, R.N., and John Machek, chaplain, with shared authority. Decisions are made by consensus. The hospice is officially part of the nonprofit, acute general hospital and is an accredited home health agency. Hospice care is provided 24 hours a day in a 10-bed unit and in the home. Services are provided to children under 16 years of age. While unit nurses are primarily responsible for home care and "on call" emergency service, they collaborate with the Visiting Nurses Association. A variable fee is charged for services. There are approximately 175,000 people in the 524 square-mile service area. Presently there are approximately 24 volunteers. Active bereavement follow-up is coordinated by Bob Fry, M.S.W. The program involves the patient's physician and pastor as important members of the care team. Major source of funding is from fees, plus contributions, and is the first hospice program approved by the Division of Health Policy and Planning of the state of Wisconsin.

CONTRIBUTORS

George J. Agich, Ph.D., is assistant professor of medical humanities and director, program in the ethics and philosophy of medicine at Southern Illinois University School of Medicine. He received his degree from the University of Texas, Austin, and was a fellow of the Institute for the Medical Humanities at The University of Texas Medical Branch, Galveston, before moving to Springfield.

Ina Ajemian, M.D., is physician-in-charge of the Palliative Care Service at The Royal Victoria Hospital in Montreal, which is a teaching hospital for McGill University. Following her internship, Dr. Ajemian acquired experience in hematology prior to a busy career in family practice. She also studied at St. Christopher's Hospice before joining the Palliative Care Unit in January 1975.

Robert W. Buckingham III, Ph.D., is former director of research and evaluation at Hospice, Inc., of New Haven, Connecticut, and now is assistant professor of health education at Teachers College, Columbia University.

James Cox, M.B., M.R.C.G.P., is chairman of the Hospice Planning Committee for St. John's Hospital in Springfield, Illinois, and assistant professor of family practice, Southern Illinois University School of Medicine. A native of England, he graduated from Newcastle-upon-Tyne Medical School in 1972 and went into general practice in Britain before moving to Springfield in 1976.

Glen W. Davidson, Ph.D., is professor and chairman, Department of Medical Humanities, professor of psychiatry and chief of thanatology, Department of Psychiatry, Southern Illinois University School of Medicine. His doctorate is from the Claremont

225

Graduate School, and he pursued postdoctoral training at The University of Chicago's and The University of Iowa's Colleges of Medicine. Before moving to Springfield, he was a member of the faculties of Colgate University and The University of Chicago, and also served as associate director of professional degrees at the latter institution. He is general editor of Augsburg's "Series On Religion and Medicine," associate editor of *Death Education: An International Quarterly,* and author of *Living With Dying,* 1975.

Richard Dayringer, Th.D., is associate professor and director of clinical education in psychosocial care, Department of Medical Humanities, and associate professor of family practice, Southern Illinois University School of Medicine. He received his doctorate from New Orleans Baptist Theological Seminary, and his clinical training at Southern Baptist Hospital in New Orleans, and Tulane University's psychiatric program at East Louisiana State Hospital, Jackson.

Parimala Desai, M.Ed., M.L.S., is director and medical librarian of St. John's Hospital, Springfield. Her degrees are from Loyola University of Chicago and the University of Oklahoma.

William C. Farr, Ph.D., M.D., is medical director of Hillhaven Hospice. He received his Ph.D. in pharmacology and his M.D. from the University of Cincinnati, is a diplomat of the American Board of Family Practice, a member of the board of directors of the Western Gerontology Society and an associate faculty member of the University of Arizona's College of Medicine.

Susan H. Foley is a master of public health candidate, Columbia University School of Public Health.

John A. Hackley, M.S.W., is president of The Hillhaven Foundation, Tacoma, Washington. Educated at Loyola University in Chicago, he was assistant director of the American Hospital Association's Division of Long Term Care before moving to Hillhaven. He is a fellow of both the American Academy of Medical Administration and the American College of Nursing Home Administrators.

Sylvia A. Lack, M.D., is medical director of Hospice, Inc., in New Haven, Connecticut. She received her degrees from London University and after her residencies became the medical officer at St. Christopher's Hospice and St. Joseph's Hospice in London. She moved to New Haven in 1973 and is known internationally for her lectures on hospice care.

William M. Lamers, Jr., M.D., is medical director and one of the founders of Hospice of Marin in California. Dr. Lamers is a psychiatrist and holds the post of assistant clinical professor of psychiatry at the University of California, San Francisco.

Theodore Raymond Leblang, J.D., is assistant professor of medical jurisprudence, director of the program in law and medicine, and associate legal counsel, Southern Illinois University School of Medicine. He is a graduate of Pennsylvania State University and the University of Illinois College of Law, and is a member of the American College of Legal Medicine.

Sr. Teresa Marie McIntier, C.S.J., is executive director of Hillhaven Hospice in Tucson. She received her training as a nurse at St. Mary's Hospital School of Nursing, Tucson, Mount St. Mary's College, Los Angeles, and her M.S.N. from the University of Arizona. She is a member of the board of directors of the Southern Arizona Cancer Society.

Balfour M. Mount, M.D., F.R.C.S., is director of the Palliative Care Unit, The Royal Victoria Hospital in Montreal. He is a graduate of Queens University and, following training as a urologist, studied at Memorial Sloan Kettering Cancer Center, New York; the Jackson Laboratory, Bar Harbor, Maine; and St. Christopher's Hospice, London. He joined the McGill University Faculty of Medicine in 1970 and is currently associate professor of surgery.

Sr. M. Simone Roach, C.S.M., Ph.D., is associate professor and chairwoman of the Department of Nursing, St. Francis Xavier University, Antigonish, Nova Scotia.

Barry Legrove Rogers, A.T.D., is director of creative communications, Hillhaven Hospice, Tucson, and a graduate student in psychology at the University of Arizona.

M. L. S. Vachon, M.A., R.N., is research scientist, Clarke Institute of Psychiatry; lecturer, Department of Psychiatry, University of Toronto; and psychiatric nurse consultant at the Princess Margaret Hospital. She received her medical training at Boston University, earned her masters degree in sociology at the University of Toronto, and is a doctoral student at York University.

Dottie C. Wilson is the coordinating administrator for the Palliative Care Service, The Royal Victoria Hospital in Montreal. She is a graduate of the University of Toronto and worked at the Massachusetts General Hospital in Boston and in private business before joining the Palliative Care Service in 1974.

Norma A. Wylie, M.Sc.N., R.N., is hospice consultant to Victoria General Hospital, Halifax, and associate professor at Dalhousie University School of Nursing. Previously, she had been a nurse educator in Singapore and Malaya for the World Health Organization, and director of nursing service at McMaster University. She is one of five Canadian nurses on The Federal Law Reform Commission's research project on protection of life.

INDEX

Administrator, 18
Admission to hospice:
    criteria for, 9, 67, 88, 135
    family involvement in, 48
    procedures in, 10
American Cancer Society, 55, 66
Antidysthanasia contract, 180-182

Barton, D., 26
Bereavement, 34
    services to survivors, 9, 12, 49,
        60, 66, 69, 84, 103
    (See also Grief)
Bowlby, J., 34
Brompton mixture, 58, 80, 91, 169
Buckingham, R., 21
Butler, R., 124

Chaplain, 16, 24, 25, 68, 71, 104,
    125
    (See also Spiritual support;
        worship service)
Clinical pharmacist, 68
Consultation, 9, 11-12, 66
Coping techniques, 121
Creative communications, 79, 125
    (See also therapeutic techniques)
Crowder, M., 26

Data Retrieval System, 137
Davidson, G. W., 32
Day care services, 66
Demographic data, 135
Dieticians, 16, 17, 68, 78

Dignity, defined, 149
Director, 17
    of creative communications, 125
Doctors (See Physicians)
Donabedian, A., 132
Drama of shock, 158

Education, 110
Education Coordinator, 18
Engel, G., 34
Epstein, C., 34
Ethics, defined, 163
Euthanasia, 174
Euthanasia Educational Council,
    178
Evaluation, 13, 19
    Buckingham model for, 130
    control group, 135
    Donabedian, model for, 131
    participant observation, 139
    practical problems, 131
    reasons for resistance to, 138
    results, 136, 139

Facilitator, 73
Family:
    anxieties, 47
    assessment of, 12
    care of, 76
    responsibilities, 10, 14, 56, 89
Feifel, H., 27, 57
Finance, 94
Fond, K. I., 77
Foucault, M., 159
Freud, S., 155-157
Fulton, R., 59

229